Contents

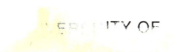
Multiple sclerosis

Sharon Warren
Professor and Director, Rehabilitation Research Centre
Faculty of Rehabilitation Medicine, University of Alberta
Edmonton, Alberta, Canada

Kenneth G. Warren
Medical Director, Multiple Sclerosis Patient Care and Research Clinic
Division of Neurology, Faculty of Medicine, University of Alberta
Edmonton, Alberta, Canada

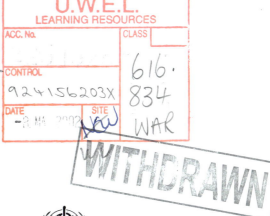

World Health Organization
Geneva
2001

WHO Library Cataloguing-in-Publication Data

Warren, Sharon
  Multiple sclerosis / Sharon Warren, Kenneth G. Warren.

  1.Multiple sclerosis 2.Risk factors I.Warren, Kenneth G. II.Title

  ISBN 92 4 156203 X   (NLM Classification: WL 360)

TYPESET IN HONG KONG
PRINTED IN MALTA
2001/13641—Best-set/Interprint—5000

Preface

As long as the etiology of multiple sclerosis remains an enigma, different approaches to its understanding are necessary. Epidemiological research has proven to be a very useful tool over recent years and dates back almost to the time when the pathological basis of the disease was described, more than 100 years ago. Epidemiology as applied to neurological disorders, and especially to such a difficult disease as multiple sclerosis, with a most often insidious onset, an unpredictable course over decades, and different prevalence rates in various geographical regions, poses particular problems of methodology. The eminent multiple sclerosis researchers Dr Sharon Warren and Dr Kenneth Warren, from Edmonton, Canada, provide an admirable overview of this difficult task by discussing, in depth and detail, the methodological aspects and results of worldwide studies, and come to considered conclusions concerning environmental and genetic factors. A separate section deals with prognostic indicators, which are often of more interest to people with multiple sclerosis than the diagnosis alone.

The publication of this monograph aptly and competently concludes the "Decade of the Brain". It includes valuable suggestions for future research that will, it is hoped, lead to a complete understanding of multiple sclerosis and eventually to the possibility of its eradication.

Professor Jürg Kesselring
Chairman, WHO Working Group on Multiple Sclerosis

1.
Introduction

Multiple sclerosis (MS) is the most common primary neurological disorder of young adults, especially in Europe and North America. The disease may affect various parts of the central nervous system (CNS), including the spinal cord, brainstem, cerebellum, cerebrum, and optic nerves, but the peripheral nerves are not affected. Pathologically, MS is characterized by numerous, discrete lesions (called plaques) scattered throughout the CNS white matter. Figure 1 shows single MS plaques in three individual patients at three different neuroanatomical sites, while Fig. 2 shows several plaques throughout the brain of one patient. The essential feature of these lesions (see Fig. 3, which shows various plaques) is loss of the myelin sheath with preservation of the axon. The presence of these lesions causes multiple, varied symptoms and signs of neurological dysfunction. One common initial symptom is optic neuritis (ON), a transient disorder of the optic nerve that often produces blurred vision or short-term blindness. Other sensory symptoms may include numbness, tingling in the hands or feet, cold or burning pain, and dizziness. Motor symptoms may include impaired coordination, imbalance, weakness, intention tremor, and spastic tone.

Not only are the symptoms of MS varied but so too is the course of the disease. In the majority of patients, symptoms occur and disappear unpredictably in its early stages, creating a relapsing–remitting (RR) disease pattern. Many patients may experience complete or partial recovery from symptoms during this phase because the axis cylinders are spared. Over time, however, symptoms may become more severe with less complete recovery of function after each exacerbation, possibly because gliosis in the margins of repeatedly affected plaques causes them to become hard or sclerotic. Patients may then enter a chronic progressive (CP) phase, characterized by a step-like downhill course.

Although some patients experience little disability during their lifetime, up to 60% are no longer fully ambulatory 20 years after onset (Weinshenker et al., 1989). Such functional decline often interferes with patients' opportunities to perform customary roles. For example, physical disability—complicated by fatigue, depression, and possibly cognitive impairment—contributes to an unemployment rate as high as 70% among patients (Scheinberg et al., 1980; LaRocca et al., 1982; Edgely, Sullivan & Dehoux, 1991). Even when patients are employed, the instability of their symptoms often results in absenteeism. Because the onset of MS is typically at about age 30,

Fig. 1. Magnetic resonance imaging of the brain of three different MS patients, illustrating start of the disease in three different anatomical areas

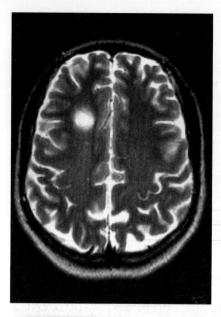

(a) An acute MS plaque in the right frontal lobe

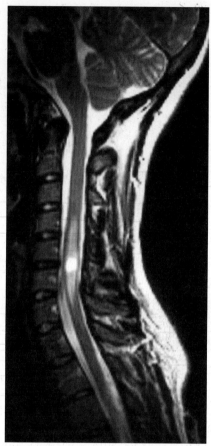

(c) An acute MS plaque in the cervical spinal cord

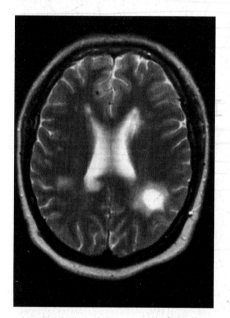

(b) An acute MS plaque in the left parietal lobe

Fig. 2. Magnetic resonance imaging (T₂ weighted) test, showing extensive bilateral acute multiple sclerosis plaques in the white matter of both parietal lobes, and fewer plaques in the frontal lobes, of a patient in a later stage of the disease

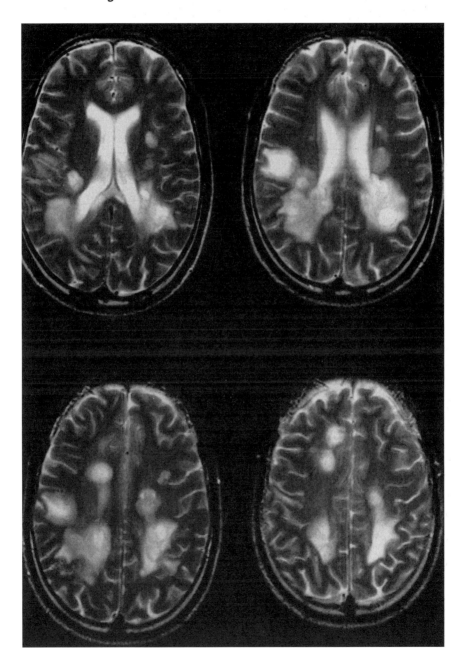

Fig. 3. Multiple sclerosis plaques

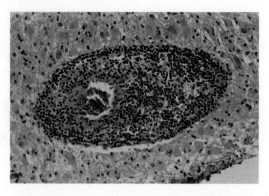

(a) Lymphocytes in the perivenular expanded Virchow–Robin space within a multiple sclerosis plaque containing macrophages

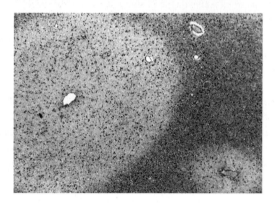

(b) Perivenular demyelination plaques with circumferential plaque borders

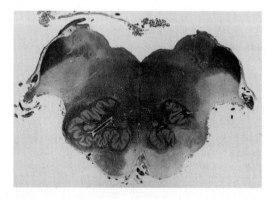

(c) Bilateral vagus nerve root entry zone plaques in the medulla oblongata, with juxtacerebrospinal fluid extension of demyelination anteriorly through the inferior olivary nucleus to the pyramidal tract on one side

patients' loss in productivity can be substantial; the financial cost to society is also great. To replace lost earnings, people with MS frequently collect disability benefits and social welfare. In addition, reports to the US National Multiple Sclerosis Society suggest that Americans with MS use more health care resources than the general population (Sternfeld, 1995). Both patients and their family members may also bear a financial burden related to home and transportation modifications, and the need for additional personal services like home-helps or child care workers. The most complete and representative cost study of MS in North America was based on 1976 data for the USA (Inman, 1984), with direct and indirect costs of MS reported for five levels of disability. Annual medical costs plus annual lost earnings at the time were estimated to total as much as US$ 15 000 per family for severely disabled patients in their prime working years. A more recent study (Harvey et al., 1994) on a non-representative population, paralysed American armed forces veterans, assessed the total annual direct plus indirect cost of MS at approximately US$ 51 000 per patient in 1992. There have also been high estimates for Canada where the Canadian Burden of Illness Study Group (1998) estimated the lifetime cost of MS, including institutionalization, to be Canadian $ 1 608 000 per patient. In North America and many other areas of the world, MS is a major public health problem.

This monograph provides a broad overview of current information on the epidemiology of MS. It begins with a discussion of diagnostic and methodological issues. Next, incidence and prevalence studies are reviewed, and differences in rates across different populations are discussed. MS risk and prognostic factors are considered, along with temporal trends in the occurrence of the disease that may provide clues to etiology. Finally, recommendations are made for future research.

who would be excluded by the rather stringent criterion of age of onset developed by Schumacher et al.

The following classification scheme, which included a formal "probable" and a "possible" category, was proposed by McAlpine (1972):

I. *Possible multiple sclerosis*
   i. Patients had an initial attack with clinical evidence of multiple lesions that suggested MS, but with unusual features or lack of signs. They had a good recovery or there was insufficient follow-up information.
   ii. Patients had a history of progressive paraplegia in early middle age without RR symptoms or a lesion outside the spinal cord. Other causes such as cervical spondylosis, spinal cord tumour and motor neuron disease were excluded by appropriate investigations.

II. *Probable multiple sclerosis*
   i. Patients had a history similar to those in category I. However, during a lengthy follow-up, they showed relative or complete absence of relapses despite a tendency towards variability in pyramidal or other signs originally present, or the appearance of an extensor plantar response, nystagmus, tremor, or temporal pallor of a disc.
   ii. Patients had a history of one or more attacks of retrobulbar neuritis accompanied or followed by usually mild pyramidal or other signs. Subsequently, they had no clinical relapses.

III. *Definite multiple sclerosis*
   i. Patients had a history of acute retrobulbar neuritis or an episode of paraesthesiae, motor weakness, double vision, unsteadiness in walking, or any other symptom associated with MS, which lessened or disappeared but was followed by one or more relapses over the years. Pyramidal and other signs indicative of multiple lesions in the CNS should have been present when patients were first seen or subsequently. Patients may not have become disabled regardless of relapses, and signs remain minimal.
   ii. Patients had experienced a gradual onset of paraplegia, later followed by relapses indicating disease in the optic nerve, cerebrum or brain stem.

McAlpine's classification system also had some limitations, particularly in the "probable" category. Patients in both subgroups of this category are expected to experience a single attack and be virtually free of relapses over a lengthy follow-up period. Patients who exhibit this pattern are relatively rare: few patients are categorized as "probable" in studies using McAlpine's classification. As for the definite category, clinicians may find it difficult to confirm reported minimal signs such as slight incoordination, absent abdominal reflexes, impaired sensation and dubious plantar reflexes. Possible MS might also be difficult to diagnose according to McAlpine's criteria, although attention to age of onset, family history, and CSF findings may help to clarify whether patients should be considered for this category. In general, the lengthy patient follow-up that is stipulated is probably not feasible for many epidemiological studies. McAlpine's classification scheme is one of the least used.

Subsequently, Rose et al. (1976) proposed an approach that combined the criteria of Schumacher et al. and McAlpine. Clinically definite (CD) MS was defined according to the relatively strict criteria of Schumacher et al., but a "probable" category similar to McAlpine's was added. Probable MS consisted of either a RR history with only one common neurological sign, or a single relapse with multifocal signs and good recovery followed by variable symptoms and signs. McDonald & Halliday (1977) also attempted to combine the criteria of Schumacher et al. with those of McAlpine, but extended the number of categories suggested by Rose et al. They accepted the Schumacher et al. criteria for CD MS, excluding progressive cases, and then added four more categories. Their "early, probable, or latent" category included patients with a single attack and evidence of multiple lesions, or patients with more than one relapse but evidence of only a single lesion. A "progressive probable" category was added for patients with progressive paraplegia plus evidence of separate lesions, while "progressive possible" included patients with evidence of only one lesion. Finally, a "suspected" category included patients who had no physical signs but had recurrent ON, with one additional episode not involving the optic nerve but without evidence of lesions outside the eye. Although McDonald & Halliday's scheme allowed for more subgroups and, like its predecessors, used fairly rigorous definitions, it did not incorporate the results of any laboratory tests to substantiate classification. Neither system has been widely used in epidemiological studies.

Bauer (1980) tried to resolve the problem of having several available diagnostic classification schemes and sought to include laboratory support of clinical classifications in some rational way. After interviewing many neurologists, he incorporated their suggestions about desirable diagnostic criteria into a new three-category system. Bauer's CD group is much the same as that used by Schumacher et al. However, to be included in the "definite" category patients must display mononuclear pleocytosis, increased gamma globulins, OCB in the gamma globulin range and evidence of immunoglobulin G (IgG) synthesis in the CNS. Bauer's "probable" and "possible" groups closely resemble those defined by McAlpine. Pathological changes in the CSF are added to the criteria for probable MS, although the full profile is not required as it is for definite cases. In the "possible" category, no CSF changes are required. In both "possible" and "probable" categories, initial attacks are included although not rigorously defined and, for the first time, monosymptomatic retrobulbar neuritis is classified as possible MS. Bauer's attempt to include laboratory tests is useful. However, if researchers apply the very rigorous definition of findings required by the "definite" category, they risk excluding some appropriate patients, since many otherwise CD- and autopsy-proven cases do not meet all of these criteria, e.g. pleocytosis. Nevertheless, Bauer's criteria have been used in a few epidemiological studies.

The latest attempt to define criteria that link clinical and laboratory findings is the diagnostic classification system of Poser et al. (1983). The system has four categories, none of which is labelled "possible":

I. *Clinically probable multiple sclerosis*
    Patients have experienced at least two relapses and show clinical evidence of one lesion; one relapse with clinical evidence of two separate lesions; or one attack with clinical evidence of one lesion and paraclinical evidence of another separate lesion.

II. *Laboratory-supported clinical multiple sclerosis*
    Patients must have had at least two attacks and CSF OCB.

III. *Clinically definite multiple sclerosis*
    Patients have had at least two relapses with clinical evidence of two separate lesions; or two relapses with clinical evidence of one and paraclinical evidence of another separate lesion.

IV. *Laboratory-supported definite multiple sclerosis*
    Patients must have had at least two relapses with either clinical or paraclinical evidence of one lesion and CSF OCB; one relapse, clinical evidence of two separate lesions, and CSF OCB; or one attack, clinical evidence of one lesion and paraclinical evidence of another separate lesion, and CSF OCB.

The criteria of Poser et al. have several advantages over previous systems. As with those of Schumacher et al., what constitutes a relapse is clearly defined, as is the number of relapses required for classification, but objective confirmation is not required and history is accepted. Paraclinical evidence, implying a lesion that has not yet produced signs and may not even have produced symptoms, is also accepted. Tests that may provide such evidence include the hot bath test, expert urological assessment, visual evoked potentials and imaging techniques. Unlike Schumacher et al., Poser et al. allow for "probable" categories that are more liberal and realistic than McAlpine's classification. The age of onset requirement of 10–59 years is also less stringent than that set by Schumacher et al. Finally, the laboratory support required by Poser et al. is more realistic than that specified by Bauer since it is confined to the presence of oligoclonal bands or increased production of IgG in the CSF. The Poser et al. classification system is the most widely used in epidemiological studies today (Rosati, 1994).

2.2 Relevance of diagnostic criteria to epidemiological research

The need for diagnostic criteria in MS is obvious, but some disagreement on both diagnosis and classification into "possible", "probable", and "definite" categories seems inevitable, regardless of whether researchers use the same or different clinical classification systems. These issues are important for epidemiological research in MS since they may influence comparisons of disease prevalence and incidence, especially when some studies include only definite cases and others incorporate probable and even possible cases.

Kurtzke (1993) has argued that, if only definite and probable cases are of interest, there should be little disagreement in the three most commonly used diagnostic classification systems—those of Allison & Millar (1954), Schumacher et al. (1965), and Poser et al. (1983). He observes that Allison & Millar's nonspecific clinical criteria are not very different from those of Schumacher et al., and that, apart from the laboratory-supported "probable" group, the categories of Poser et al. can be made to fit these earlier classification systems.

Unfortunately, few published studies have formally addressed the reliability and validity of the various diagnostic classification systems. A study from the United Kingdom (Mumford et al., 1992) at least partially supports Kurtzke's contention. Using the Allison & Millar criteria, Mumford et al. reported a prevalence rate (excluding "possibles") of 107 in Cambridge, while Swingler & Compston (1988) reported a rate of 84 in South Glamorgan and Roberts et al. (1991) a rate of 92 in Southampton. Using the criteria of Poser et al., Mumford et al. (1992) reported rates of 112, 101, and 95 in the same three regions. For Cambridge and Southampton the differences are minimal, but prevalence for South Glamorgan based on the Poser et al. criteria is considerably higher than prevalence based on Allison & Millar. On the other hand, Palffy (1988) has shown that the use of Bauer's criteria and those of Schumacher et al. might produce different numbers in epidemiological studies. Using a large autopsy series, Palffy compared the diagnostic value of these two classification systems. For Bauer's criteria, both sensitivity and specificity were 1.0, while for those of Schumacher et al. the values were 0.76 and 0.68 respectively, implying that Bauer's criteria had the superior predictive value. Rosati (1994) pointed out that use of less stringent diagnostic criteria alone might produce higher rates in some regions than use of more stringent criteria.

Even when the same classification system is used, it may produce different numbers. Hammond et al. (1988a) examined the inter-rater reliability of the Rose et al. classification system. An independent rater assessed a 10% sample of patients from three Australian cities (Perth, Newcastle, and Hobart). While there was little disagreement on the diagnosis of MS, there was some variation in the level of agreement on diagnostic classification ("definite" versus "probable"): the independent assessment agreed with the classification in 70%, 94%, and 80% of cases respectively across the three centres. In studies that use only definite cases, or that calculate separate rates for definite and probable MS, such disagreement might lead to differences in numbers from one region to another, although it is noteworthy that the level of disagreement in the three Australian cities was not statistically significant.

Some increases in the incidence and prevalence of MS within the same region may also be due to modified application of the same test. For example, an epidemiological study in Groningen, Netherlands, showed an increase in prevalence from 50/100 000 population in 1981 to 76/100 000 in 1992, and an increase in annual incidence from 2/100 000 before 1985 to 6/100 000 between 1985 and 1992 (Prange et al., 1986). The Poser et al. criteria were used for both data collection periods, but MRI was used more frequently to supplement the diagnostic procedure after 1985. The extent to which such techniques are used varies from country to country: they are less likely to be used in developing countries and eastern Europe than in western Europe or North America, which might produce a different impression of current rates or rate changes from one region to another.

A further issue to be kept in mind when comparing prevalence and incidence rates is whether researchers permit the inclusion of Devic syndrome or other demyelinating disease, as Japanese and other east Asian groups do (Kuroiwa et al., 1982). C.M. Poser (1994) suggests that patients with Devic syndrome should be included only rarely as cases of MS. He recommends criteria for their inclusion: a period of 6 months must have elapsed between the optic and myelic components, or evidence of a new, separate lesion must appear indicating involvement of the brain. Poser also recommends the use of MRI to avoid misclassifying multiphasic disseminated encephalomyelitis as MS, since the two are clinically indistinguishable. He points out that criteria for better differentiation of MS from other conditions such as chronic fatigue syndrome, Lyme disease, and HTLV-1-associated paraparesis need to be developed.

2.3 Case-ascertainment methods

In the past, the frequency of MS was inferred from mortality reports based on death certificates kept by various countries and published by the World Health Organization. Coding is based on definitions in the *International Statistical Classification of Diseases and Related Health Problems*, now in its tenth revision (ICD-10). The ICD-10 classification for MS is shown in Table 1. Mortality data are subject to misdiagnosis and coding error even when the ICD definitions or other criteria are being used. In addition, death certificates may not list the presence of a disease unless it is the cause of death. Mortality reports may accurately indicate the frequency of diseases that lead to severe disability with short survival, since the diagnosis is usually listed as the primary or secondary cause of death. However, the course of MS may be relatively benign with long survival, and death in about 50% of cases is due to some other disease (Leibowitz et al., 1972). For this reason, MS may not be mentioned at all in death certificates or, if mentioned, not listed as a cause of death. For example, Kahana & Zilber (1996) found that 435 Israeli MS Registry patients died between 1955 and 1985, but that MS was mentioned as the primary cause of death of only 24% and not mentioned at all on the death certificates of 32% of patients.

Table 1. ICD-10 classification for multiple sclerosis[a]

G35	**Multiple sclerosis**
	Includes: multiple sclerosis (of)
	• NOS[b]
	• brain stem
	• cord
	• disseminated
	• generalized
	Excludes: concentric sclerosis [Baló] (G37.5)
	neuromyelitis optica [Devic] (G36.0)
	Note: These conditions are classified to other ICD-10 categories even if they are often considered as variants of multiple sclerosis.
G35.–0	Relapsing/remitting multiple sclerosis
G35.–1	Primary progressive multiple sclerosis
	Chronic progressive multiple sclerosis, progressive from onset
G35.–2	Secondary progressive multiple sclerosis
	Chronic progressive multiple sclerosis, after an initially relapsing/remitting course (includes remittent progressive)
G35.–8	Other symptomatic forms of multiple sclerosis

[a] Extracted from *Application of the International Classification of Diseases to Neurology*, 2nd ed. Geneva, World Health Organization, 1997.
[b] not otherwise specified.

More recently, the frequency of MS has been described on the basis of research conducted specifically to assess its incidence and prevalence in various countries and using one of the diagnostic classification systems outlined in section 2.1. The accuracy of MS incidence and prevalence rates in such studies is influenced not only by the diagnostic criteria applied but also by case-ascertainment methods. Several approaches to case-ascertainment can be used in epidemiological studies.

The most accurate approach is the door-to-door survey, using skilled clinicians to examine suspected cases in order to arrive at a diagnosis according to standardized criteria and to ascertain that onset of a condition has occurred. Such MS studies have been conducted in a number of locations, for example in Sicily (Meneghini et al., 1991). However, because of the human resources necessary, this approach is feasible only for small communities in geographically limited areas. It is also complicated by the low frequency of MS in particular areas: studies of this type usually produce small numbers of cases and rates with wide confidence intervals (CIs).

A more common approach is to count new or existing cases seen at treatment facilities within a given study area. The accuracy of this approach depends on the range and number of facilities used. Ideally all facilities from a wide range of possibilities should be used, including general hospitals, long-term care facilities, neurology and general practice clinics, and specialized MS clinics. Even then, the accuracy of case-finding depends on how many patients actually come to the attention of the researchers and on the quality of each facility's record-keeping system.

The percentage of MS patients seen at treatment facilities may vary from country to country. It is higher in countries where most of the population is covered by prepaid medical insurance and where most MS patients may therefore be seen in hospital at some point. Kahana & Zilber (1996) have reported that in Israel, where 90% of the population are covered by insurance, 94% of MS patients are hospitalized within 10 years of disease onset and 77% within 5 years. In countries where fewer people are insured these figures are likely to be lower. Hospital admission rates also vary between and within countries according to hospital policy, producing different impressions of disease frequency. The exclusive use of hospital files as sources of data may also result in the under-representation of less severe cases across studies.

Similarly, not all individuals with MS may be seen at neurology outpatient clinics, by private neurologists, in general practice, or even in specialized MS clinics. Throughout Canada there are a number of MS clinics associated with university hospitals. However, in an MS prevalence study of Barrhead County, Alberta (Warren & Warren, 1992), only 15 of 21 patients identified by various sources had been seen in the Multiple Sclerosis Patient Care and Research Clinic at the University of Alberta although it was readily accessible to all patients.

A universal problem with the use of treatment facility files is that there may be no specific statement of diagnosis or of a diagnostic code such as the ICD-10 code. For example, Kahana & Zilber (1996) found that, out of 23 Israeli hospitals, only two in Jerusalem had outpatient clinics that used a coded diagnostic index. The files kept by neurologists and general practitioners in private practice are equally lacking in such detail, if not more so. To complicate matters, hospital facilities or private practices that use diagnostic codes may not have computerized data systems available, making it necessary for researchers to read and interpret all records. The quality of medical records also varies widely in Europe. Italian hospitals, particularly in the centre and south of the country, lack computer-based hospital systems, as do many facilities in some regions of Greece, Portugal, and Spain, and probably many areas of eastern Europe (Rosati, 1994). Defined diagnostic criteria may not be consistently applied across facilities within or among regions in which epidemiological studies have been conducted.

Special "case registries" are the basis of another approach to identifying MS patients. Registries like the Danish Multiple Sclerosis Registry (Koch-Henriksen & Hyllested, 1988), which was established in 1948, are rare. Several possible sources of patients provide information to the Registry, including neurological departments of Danish hospitals, treatment centres of the MS Society, the National Patient Registry (all hospital patients), and the National Registry of Causes of Death. The completeness of such registries also depends on the range and number of referral sources and, in turn, on the completeness of the records maintained by those sources.

In some countries where health care is publicly funded, government recording systems have been used to estimate the frequency of MS. Svenson, Woodhead & Platt (1994) used Alberta (Canada) Health Care Insurance Plan records to identify patients whose physician billings indicated a diagnosis of MS according to the classification in the ninth revision of ICD (ICD-9). Reluctance on the part of physicians to diagnose MS without a fair degree of certainty may mean that, although most patients so billed to Alberta Health are likely to have MS, some suspected or possible cases might not be recorded. However, Svenson, Woodhead & Platt found a high correlation between rates generated through health insurance plan records and those reported by independent community surveys conducted in selected Alberta census divisions.

Another possible source of patients is MS society records. A small number of patients registered in MS society rosters do not fit standard diagnostic criteria (Anderson et al., 1992). However, many patients do not register with MS societies because they do not want to acknowledge or publicize their condition or be in contact with other patients perhaps more disabled than themselves.

Finally, in certain instances, identification of cases may be based on information provided by selected key informants with wide social contacts and an intimate knowledge of the community. This technique would be useful for studying MS among groups living a somewhat self-contained existence within developed countries (such as the Hutterites in Canada) or in certain areas of the developing world, but is not suitable in large industrialized regions where residents generally know only a limited number of other community members.

Each of these case-finding methods has strengths and weaknesses. Epidemiological research may require a combination of approaches to maximize accuracy.

3.
Epidemiology of multiple sclerosis

The incidence and prevalence of MS have been studied extensively. Some features of the disease are generally accepted:

- The frequency of MS varies by geographical region throughout the world, apparently increasing with distance from the Equator in both hemispheres.
- The disease is more common among women than men.
- Peak onset is around age 30 years.
- The disease is less common among non-white individuals than whites.

The distributions of MS by geography, sex, age, and race or ethnicity have all been explored for clues to etiology. Most early research focused on the possible role of an environmental factor that varied with latitude. To date no such risk factor for the disease has been unequivocally identified, although researchers continue to believe that one exists. There is substantial evidence of a genetic predisposition to the disease based on familial aggregation, and some debate over whether genetics or exposure to an environmental trigger primarily accounts for its geographical distribution. Relatively little is known about factors that predict the course of MS.

3.1 Appropriate use of incidence and prevalence rates to study etiology

Although most epidemiologists agree that the frequency of MS differs throughout geographical regions of the world, many question the extent of such variation and how it should be interpreted when exploring etiology. The debate about the extent of variations in frequency is largely focused on methodological issues surrounding the estimation of incidence and prevalence rates. However, the biological relevance of these rates must also be kept in mind when any attempt is made to identify potential causal factors.

3.1.1 Methodological issues affecting the comparison of rates among geographical areas

Incidence and prevalence rates are different, but the methodological issues affecting their accuracy are similar. Incidence is defined as the number of new cases occurring (numerator) in a given population during a specified time period (denominator). For MS, this is usually a 5–10-year period because of the low occurrence of the disease. Unlike incidence, which focuses on onset, prevalence focuses on disease status. Prevalence is defined as the number of existing cases of a disease (numerator) in a given population on a particular date or during a specified time period (denominator). Prevalence rates reflect not only the occurrence but also the duration of a condition. According to Kramer's (1957) formula, prevalence is approximately equal to incidence multiplied by the average duration in years of the disease. MS is an example of a chronic disease with low incidence but long average duration and low case-fatality, so that its prevalence is relatively high compared with its incidence. The determination of numerator and denominator is problematic for both rates and subject to biases, as discussed below.

Incidence and prevalence rates in many MS studies are based on small numbers of cases because of the low frequency of the disease. Diagnostic criteria and case-ascertainment methods can affect the number of cases identified and account for differences in rates between one geographical region and another. The omission of even a few patients from the numerator can lead to serious underestimation of rates. For example, a survey in Westlock County, Alberta, Canada, identified 23 patients with probable or definite MS in a population of 11 510 and gave a prevalence rate of 200/100 000 (Warren & Warren, 1993). If only one of these patients had been missed, the prevalence rate would have been 191/100 000.

Errors in the size of the denominator, resulting from problems such as inaccuracies in census data, are less likely to influence rates than is failure to identify cases of MS. However, when disease rates in different populations are compared, other considerations regarding the denominator can be important. Since MS prevalence is influenced by disease duration, apparent differences in rates between geographical regions may be partially explained by regional differences in medical intervention. In addition, different populations should be examined to determine whether their profiles differ with respect to factors such as age, sex, and race or ethnicity, which affect occurrence of MS. For instance, a lower MS prevalence rate has been observed in the northern counties of Troms and Finnmark, Norway, than in the rest of the country, but has partially been explained by the higher percentage of Lapps (who apparently do not acquire MS) in that area (Koch-Henriksen, 1995).

To minimize bias in comparing rates between populations that differ with regard to such factors, crude rates should be standardized (Lilienfeld & Stolley, 1994). In this procedure, a hypothetical crude rate—based on the weighted average of category-specific rates taken from a standard distribution—is calculated for each population to be compared. In essence, rates for different populations are reduced to a common denominator so that they can be compared without confounding by the variable on which they have been standardized. An example would be age standardization based on the age structure of the population of the USA. Age is a typical consideration in MS since onset is most commonly in the late 20s and 30s; unfortunately, there is no general agreement on the standard that should be used in adjusting for this factor. Moreover, there is often no information available on the structure of various populations according to race or ethnicity, so that standardization on this factor, which may often account for differences in the geographical frequency of MS, is impossible.

Both incidence and prevalence rates for MS are subject to sampling error, which means that their estimates in the population will vary from sample to sample, even if samples are selected randomly from the entire population. The confidence interval—a range of possible values—should be calculated for observed rates. The width of CIs will vary with two factors: the variability in the data and the level of confidence desired for the range. A small number of cases in the numerator means higher variability in the data; the calculated rate will consequently be less precise and its CI wide. CIs should be calculated using the Poisson probability distribution, suitable for situations in which the numerator is small and the denominator is large (Rothman, 1986). Usually the CI is set at 95%, so that there is a 95% chance that the true population rate falls somewhere in the calculated range.

Confidence intervals can be used to determine whether the differences in rates observed in various populations are significantly different. In general, if the 95% CIs for two rates do not overlap, the 95% CI calculated for the difference between them would not include 0; in other words the rates are different. On the other hand, if the 95% CIs do overlap, the rates are not necessarily the same. The 95% CI associated with the difference between them should be calculated, unless the 95% CI for one rate includes the actual value of the other rate. In this instance, the 95% CI for the rate difference will usually include 0; that is, the rate in the two populations is the same.

There is a trade-off between studying small populations, which may be expected to produce only a small number of MS cases, and studying larger populations, which are likely to produce larger numbers. Diagnostic criteria can be more tightly controlled and case-ascertainment more thorough in small, intensively studied areas. Underestimation can be a problem when very large populations are studied under less than optimal conditions. Because MS registers like that in Denmark are rare, investigators must typically rely on physicians, clinics, or hospital records as their sources of information. Rosati (1994) has suggested that rates calculated from recent large-scale studies in eastern Europe and the former Soviet Union are probably underestimates because of the more poorly organized medical systems in those regions. In addition, rather unremarkable differences in rates between large populations can generate highly significant P values.

3.1.2 Biological relevance of prevalence versus incidence

There is no doubt that prevalence studies can be useful in establishing the need for health services. However, they have also been used to generate hypotheses about etiological factors, which is a questionable practice. Besides the methodological issues that may complicate comparisons between regions, the biological relevance of prevalence rates must be addressed. Since the prevalence rate is based on cases existing within a geographical region at a given point in time, it may include people who experienced the onset of MS before immigrating to the area—in other words, people who were exposed to an environmental risk factor elsewhere. Prevalence rates are thus potentially misleading. For example, a risk factor may be more common in several rural areas adjacent to a large city than in the city itself. If patients move from rural areas to the city, once they acquire the disease, in order to have access to better medical facilities, there would be no correlation between the prevalence rate and the etiological factor because the one will be high where the other is low. Consequently, when prevalence rates are used to explore etiology, they should at least be adjusted to exclude people who acquired the disease outside the areas being compared. Such rates may be substantially lower if affected immigrants are excluded.

Rates calculated for Olmsted County, Minnesota, USA, in 1978 illustrate the impact of excluding immigrants on prevalence rates (Kranz et al., 1983). Of the 91 patients identified, giving a prevalence rate of 102/100 000, 25 had moved to the county after onset of symptoms. The prevalence rate based only on residents, who had experienced the onset of MS symptoms within the county, was 74/100 000. Unfortunately, many studies do not make such adjustments, nor do they provide the information from which readers could calculate adjusted rates.

The use of incidence rates to explore etiology would be preferable. Incidence rates inherently have more biological relevance because they represent new cases occurring within a given area during some period of time. However, their use is complicated by other factors, including the methodological issues that influence prevalence rates and the fact that they are so low. In addition, onset is notoriously difficult to pinpoint. Identification of onset is frequently based on patient recall of symptoms, which may be unreliable; early symptoms may be too mild to have been noticed or to warrant being counted by a clinician even if they are reported. Date of diagnosis, although more clear cut, is not an appropriate substitute for onset when exploring etiology because the lag time from onset to diagnosis may vary with the willingness or ability of clinicians to label early cases. If a risk factor is high during a period when many individuals present with symptoms to physicians but declines during the lag time between first appearance of symptoms and actual diagnosis, any correlation between the risk factor and onset will be masked if date of diagnosis is used as a proxy for onset.

It is possible that neither onset of symptoms nor diagnosis accurately reflects acquisition of the disease, since migration studies indicate that some environmental risk factor operates before age 15 years, yet onset peaks around age 30 (Kurtzke, 1985). Given this long latency period, patients may well be living somewhere different when they first experience symptoms from where they were living when they acquired the disease. Incidence rates probably reflect clinical manifestation of the disease rather than acquisition, and factors correlated with each event may differ. In any investigation of factors related to etiology, the comparison of incidence rates among geographical regions may therefore be misleading, just as prevalence rates are. If incidence rates are used for this purpose, they should ideally be based only on people who have lived more or less all their lives (or at least until age 15) in the comparison areas. With current population mobility in many areas of the world, this stipulation is probably unrealistic.

3.2 Prevalence and incidence of multiple sclerosis worldwide

Numerous prevalence studies provide a detailed picture of the geographical distribution of MS, but more of these pertain to the northern than to the southern hemisphere. Incidence studies generally support the distribution observed in prevalence studies. Not only has prevalence been shown to vary with latitude, but migration studies have also demonstrated that risk can be altered by change of residence, and both geographical and temporal clusters of MS have been documented. Sex-, age-, and race-specific rates, however, exhibit similar patterns in both high- and low-risk areas.

3.2.1 Prevalence rates

The uneven geographical distribution of MS has been recognized for over 75 years. After the First World War, Davenport (1922) observed a higher frequency of the disease among American armed forces veterans drafted from the Great Lakes, and from Washington and other northern states than among those from the southern states. Several years later Steiner (1938) was the first to propose that the occurrence of MS was associated with geographical factors, and Ulett (1946) suggested that high MS frequency was associated with northern latitudes. The earliest analysis of the distribution of MS was conducted by Limburg (1950) who used mortality rates to infer prevalence; he observed that mortality was higher among countries in temperate zones than in the tropics. He also noted higher rates in northern Italy and the northern USA than in the southernmost parts of those countries. Later studies (Goldberg & Kurland, 1962; Massey & Schoenburg, 1982) found that MS death rates for all countries were lower than in earlier studies, but their ranking was quite similar to Limburg's. The highest rates found by Goldberg & Kurland were in Ireland and Scotland (3.1 and 3.0 per 100 000, respectively). Other western European countries generally had high rates, except in the northernmost parts of Finland, Norway, and Sweden and in Greece and Italy, where rates were classified as medium. Rates in Australia, Canada, New Zealand, and the USA were comparable to the medium or higher rates found in western Europe. The lowest rates by far (0.1, 0.1, and 0 per 100 000) were found in Japan, South Africa, and the Philippines, respectively.

Since the Second World War, more than 300 studies of the worldwide prevalence of MS have been reported; the results of many of these are summarized in Table 2. In reviewing the rates presented it is important to remember that:

- The studies from which they are derived may vary in terms of both diagnostic criteria (especially the inclusion of "possible" and "probable" patients) and case-ascertainment methods.
- Some rates may be crude while others are adjusted (most likely for age).
- Apparently substantial differences from one place to another might disappear if CIs were applied.
- Some frequency studies were conducted in large, heavily populated areas whereas others were carried out in circumscribed, less populated areas.

Nevertheless, these studies generally confirm the pattern observed in those based on mortality statistics—the frequency of MS increases with distance from the Equator.

Prevalence surveys conducted in the northern hemisphere before 1980 suggested a steady progression of risk, with some flattening and increased scatter by latitude 50°N (Acheson, 1985). This progression was observed not only between countries such as those of western Europe (Kurtzke, 1980) but also within the USA (Kurtzke, Beebe & Norman, 1979) and within the United Kingdom as a whole (Forbes & Swingler, 1999); this was not true, however, within either England (Ford et al., 1998) or Scotland alone (Grant, Carver & Sloan, 1998; Rothwell & Charlton, 1998; Forbes, Wilson & Swingler, 1999). Fewer studies of the southern hemisphere are available, but surveys from Australia (McCall et al., 1968) and New Zealand (Acheson, 1961) indicated a similar latitude pattern. On the basis of the pattern observed in these studies, epidemiologists initially tended to divide the world into zones of high, medium and low MS risk. The ranges most frequently quoted define high prevalence as more than 30 cases per 100 000 population, medium as 5–29 per 100 000, and low as 0–4 per 100 000 (Kurtzke, 1980).

Surveys in southern Europe since 1980 have diminished the concept of a north–south gradient in the northern hemisphere. Whereas before 1980 prevalence rates in southern Europe were considered to range from 5 to 29 per 100 000, more recent studies in southern France, Greece, Italy, and Spain have produced rates averaging about 50 per 100 000 (Rosati, 1994). Some researchers (for example, C.M. Poser, 1994) have argued that these countries should be reclassified as high risk and that the commonly accepted north–south gradient in Europe has lost its credibility. Others, including Lauer (1994), contend that the ranges for low, medium, and high should simply be revised upwards, since the most recent studies in north–western Europe have also produced prevalence rates that are both higher than those derived from earlier studies

Table 2. Prevalence rates for multiple sclerosis[a]

Country and/or region	Latitude	Year	Prevalence per 100 000 pop.	References
Norway				
Troms and Finmark	68°N	1983	31	Grønning & Mellgren (1985)
More and Romsdal	63°N	1985	75	Midgard, Riise & Nyland (1994)
Hordaland	60°N	1983	60	Larsen et al. (1984a)
Iceland (all)	63–66°N	1989	92	Benedikz et al. (1994)
Russian Federation				
Siberia	65°N	1994	12	Boiko et al. (1995)
Novgorod	58°N	1994	36	Boiko et al. (1995)
Moscow	55°N	1994	32	Boiko et al. (1995)
Kchabarovsk	48°N	1994	41	Boiko et al. (1995)
Stavropol	45°N	1994	24	Boiko et al. (1995)
Finland				
Vaasa	63°N	1979	93	Kinnunen et al. (1983)
Uusimaa	60°N	1979	52	Kinnunen et al. (1983)
Denmark (all)	54–62°N	1965	101	Bauer (1987)
Faeroe Islands	62°N	1977	34	Kurtzke & Hyllested (1979)
United Kingdom				
Scotland				
Orkney Islands	60°N	1983	224	Cook et al. (1985)
Shetland Islands	60°N	1984	170	Cook et al. (1988)
Aberdeen	57°N	1980	144	Phadke & Downie (1987)
Grampian region	57°N	1980	145	Phadke & Downie (1987)
Outer Hebrides	57°N	1979	97	Dean, Goodall & Downie (1981)
England				
Northumberland	55°N	1958	42	Poskanzer, Schapira & Miller (1963a)
Cambridge	52°N	1990	112	Mumford et al. (1992)
Sutton (London borough)	51°N	1985	104	Williams & McKeran (1986)
Cornwall	51°N	1958	63	Hargreaves (1969)
Southampton	50°N	1987	95	Roberts et al. (1990)
Sussex	50°N	1991	111	Rice-Oxley, Williams & Rees (1995)
Channel Islands				
Jersey	49–50°N	1991	113	Sharpe et al. (1995)
Guernsey	49–50°N	1991	87	Sharpe et al. (1995)
Northern Ireland	55°N	1954	41	Allison & Millar (1954)
Wales				
Glamorgan, south	51°N	1985	101	Swingler & Compston (1988)
Sweden				
Gothenburg	58°N	1988	96	Svenningsson et al. (1990)
Estonia (south)	57–59°N	1988–1989	51	Gross, Kokk & Kaasik (1993)
Pôlva County	58°N	1988–1989	72	Gross, Kokk & Kaasik (1993)
Tartu	58°N	1988–1989	31	Gross, Kokk & Kaasik (1993)
Jôgeva	58°N	1988–1989	40	Gross, Kokk & Kaasik (1993)
Viljandi	58°N	1988–1989	40	Gross, Kokk & Kaasik (1993)
Vôru	58°N	1988–1989	59	Gross, Kokk & Kaasik (1993)
Valga	57°N	1988–1989	58	Gross, Kokk & Kaasik (1993)
Germany				
Hamburg	54°N	1960	57	Behrend (1966)
Rostock	54°N	1983	67	Meyer-Rienecker (1994)
Stralsund/Rügen	54°N	1988	62	Meyer-Rienecker (1994)
Halle	52°N	1984	43	Schmidt et al. (1989)

Table 2. Continued

Country and/or region	Latitude	Year	Prevalence per 100 000 pop.	References
Bochum	52°N	1990	95	Haupts et al. (1994)
Lower Saxony (south)	51–52°N	1992	108	S. Poser (1994)
Hesse (south)	49–50°N	1992	85	Lauer & Firnhaber (1994)
Darmstadt	50°N	1982	54	Prange et al. (1986)
Poland				
Szczecin	54°N	1992	62	Potemkowski et al. (1994)
Western region	52–53°N	1981	43	Wender et al. (1985)
Canada				
British Columbia	54°N	1982	117	Sweeney, Sadovnick & Brandejs (1986)
Barrhead County, Alberta	54°N	1990	196	Warren & Warren (1992)
Westlock County, Alberta	54°N	1991	200	Warren & Warren (1993)
Cardston, Alberta	49°N	1989	87	Klein, Rose & Seland (1994)
Crowsnest Pass, Alberta	49°N	1989	202	Klein, Rose & Seland (1994)
Saskatoon, Saskatchewan	52°N	1999	248	Hader (1999)
Winnipeg, Manitoba	50°N	1960	35	Stazio et al. (1964)
Ottawa, Ontario	45°N	1975	67	Bennett et al. (1976)
Kingston, Ontario	44°N	1941	30	White & Wheelan (1959)
London, Ontario	43°N	1984	94	Hader, Elliot & Ebers (1988)
Halifax, Nova Scotia	45°N	1960	25	Alter et al. (1960)
Newfoundland	52°N	1985	55	Pryse-Phillips (1986)
Netherlands				
Groningen	53°N	1982	54	Prange et al. (1986)
Czech Republic				
Bohemia (north-west)	51°N	1992	89	Jedlicka et al. (1994)
Bohemia (east)	51°N	1984	51	Jedlicka (1989)
Prague	50°N	1984	67	Bauer (1987)
Belgium (all)	49–52°N	1983	80–100	Bauer (1987)
Flanders	50°N	1983	74	Van Ooteghem et al. (1994)
Austria				
(Upper/Lower)	46–48°N	1972	29/22	Bauer (1987)
Vienna	48°N	1972	42	Bauer (1987)
France				
Brittany	48°N	1978	25	Gallou et al. (1983)
Chalon-sur-Naon	46°N	1984	58	Confavreux et al. (1987)
Arles	44°N	1980	9	Poser (1994)
Avignon	43°N	1984	49	Confavreux et al. (1987)
Pyrénées-Atlantiques	43°N	1988	38	Roth et al. (1994)
Marseilles	43°N	1960	14	Behrend et al. (1963)
Romania				
34 counties	43–48°N	1984	26	Petrescu (1994)
Cluj, Transylvania	46°N	1984	43	Bauer (1987)
Brasov, Transylvania	45°N	1984	46	Bauer (1987)
Danube (southern regions)	45°N	1984	<6	Bauer (1987)
Bucharest	44°N	1984	79	Bauer (1987)
Switzerland (all)	46–48°N	1986	52	Kesselring & Beer (1994)
Berne	47°N	1986	110	Kesselring & Beer (1994)
Basel	47°N	1984	170	Groebke-Lorenz et al. (1992)
Valais	46°N	1977	25	Bartschi-Rochaix (1980)

Table 2. Continued

Country and/or region	Latitude	Year	Prevalence per 100 000 pop.	References
China				
Lan Cang La Hu Zu (Yunnan)	24–26°N	1986	2	Hou & Zhang (1992)
China (Province of Taiwan)	23°N	1975	1	Hung (1982)
Hong Kong Special Adminstrative Region of China	22°N	1987	0.9	Yu et al. (1989)
India				
Bombay	19°N	1988	26	Wadia & Bhatia (1990)
Poona	18°N	1988	58	Wadia & Bhatia (1990)
Malaysia	2°N	1986	2	Tan (1988)
Peru				
Lima	12°S	1974	5	Kurtzke (1980)
Australia				
Queensland	15–27°S	1981	18	Hammond et al. (1987)
Perth, WA	32°S	1981	30	Hammond et al. (1988a)
Adelaide, SA	32°S	1981	32	McLeod, Hammond & Hallpike (1994)
Newcastle, NSW	33°S	1981	37	Hammond et al. (1988a)
Hobart, Tas.	43°S	1981	76	Hammond et al. (1988a)
Brazil				
São Paulo	24°S	1990	4	Callegaro et al. (1992)
South Africa (whites)	30°S	1960	11	Dean (1967)
Argentina				
Buenos Aires	34°S	1974	15	Kurtzke (1980)
New Zealand				
Waikata region, N. Island	39°S	1981	24	Skegg et al. (1987)
Wellington	41°S	1968	39	Hornabrook (1971)
Christchurch	43°S	1972	37	Cunningham (1972)
Otago region, S. Island	43°S	1981	69	Skegg et al. (1987)

[a] Country names used in this table are those that are valid at the time of publication of this book.

and are still, on average, higher than those for southern Europe. Nevertheless, most epidemiologists would agree that the north–south gradient in Europe seems less steep than it did in the past.

The geographical pattern of MS within the northern hemisphere also shows striking variations at the same latitudes, both between and within countries and within sub-regions of countries. For example, Olmsted County in Minnesota, USA, and Arles in France are at virtually the same latitude (44°N) but have prevalence rates of 122 and 9 per 100 000 respectively. Rates within Germany range from 43 to 108 per 100 000, and in Italy from 33 in L'Aquila on the mainland to 103 per 100 000 in the north–west of Sardinia. Within the province of Newfoundland, Canada, prevalence varies from 16 to 105 per 100 000 (Pryse-Phillips, 1986) and within the Canton of Berne in Switzerland from 65 to 154 per 100 000 (Beer & Kesselring, 1994).

The north–south gradient originally observed in the southern hemisphere has been confirmed by new studies and is less debatable. Two surveys in Australia, 30 years apart, have both demonstrated that prevalence of MS in Hobart, Tasmania, is twice that in the cities of Perth and Newcastle in southern Australia (McLeod, Hammond & Hallpike, 1994). Although there have been few carefully conducted studies in Africa, India, South America, and south-east Asia, MS prevalence in these areas seems to be uniformly low, regardless of latitude.

3.2.2 Incidence rates

Because the time of onset of MS, unlike many diseases, is difficult to define and subject to considerable inaccuracy, there have been fewer studies of incidence of the disease than of its prevalence. Table 3 summarizes several of the studies conducted to date. The same considerations apply to a geographical comparison of incidence rates as to a comparison of prevalence rates: in general, incidence rates parallel prevalence rates. The highest rates in the northern hemisphere are found in Scotland and the lowest in the southern USA (New Orleans). Rates in Israel and Japan are also thought to be low, at less than 1 per 100 000 population. Again, recent studies in southern Europe have diminished the idea of a north–south incidence gradient in the northern hemisphere and have revealed striking variations in incidence within countries. For example, Aberdeen, Scotland, and Gothenburg, Sweden, which are at virtually the same latitude (58°N), have reported incidence rates of 7.2 and 2.6 per 100 000 respectively. Rates range from 1.9 to 5.5 per 100 000 within Norway, from 0.8 to 3.2 per 100 000 within Hungary, and from 2.2 in Ferrara on mainland Italy to 7.5 per 100 000 in Alghero, Sardinia.

Incidence in the southern hemisphere has been less well studied, but it is thought to be uniformly low except in Australia and New Zealand. The highest reported rate is for Newcastle, Australia, and the lowest for South Africa (among native-born individuals).

3.2.3 Migration studies

Many studies have concentrated on migration between areas with different MS prevalence rates: any evidence that migration affects risk would tend to substantiate the involvement of an environmental geographical factor. Ideally, migrant studies should be based on the incidence of MS among immigrants *after* arrival in a new country, so that it is at least clear where the onset of symptoms was first experienced, if not where the disease was acquired. However, because of the generally low occurrence of the condition, most studies have compared the prevalence of MS among immigrants with that among native-born residents of the new country or with prevalence in the immigrants' place of origin.

Table 3. Average annual incidence rates for multiple sclerosis[a]

Country and/or region	Latitude	Period	Incidence per 100 000 pop.	References
Norway				
Troms and Finmark	68°N	1974–1982	1.9	Grønning & Mellgren (1985)
More and Romsdal	63°N	1985–1991	5.5	Midgard, Riise & Nyland (1994)
Hordaland	60°N	1973–1982	2.4	Larsen et al. (1984b)
Iceland (all)	63–66°N	1975–1985	2.7	Poser, Benedikz & Hibberd (1992)
Finland				
Vaasa	63°N	1969–1978	3.3	Kinnunen (1984)
Uusimaa	60°N	1969–1978	2.3	Kinnunen (1984)
United Kingdom				
Scotland				
Orkney Islands	60°N	1940–1982	8.9	Cook et al. (1985)
Shetland Islands	60°N	1940–1986	7.2	Cook et al. (1988)
Aberdeen	57°N	1977–1980	7.2	Phadke & Downie (1987)
Grampian Region	57°N	1960–1980	5.9	Phadke & Downie (1987)
England				
Cambridge	52°N	1989–1991	5.9	Mumford et al. (1992)
Sutton (London borough)	51°N	1974–1984	5.0	Williams & McKeran (1986)
Southampton	50°N	1976–1982	4.7	Roberts et al. (1990)
Northern Ireland	55°N	1985–1992	6.5	McDonnell & Hawkins (1998)
Sweden				
Gothenburg	58°N	1974–1988	2.6	Svenningsson et al. (1990)
Denmark	54–58°N	1978–1987	4.8	Koch-Henriksen et al. (1994)
Germany				
Rostock	54°N	1974–1983	2.8	Meyer-Rienecker (1994)
Stralsund/Rügen	54°N	1979–1987	1.9	Meyer-Rienecker (1994)
Halle	52°N	1970–1984	2.0	Schmidt et al. (1989)
Lower Saxony (south)	51–52°N	1970–1985	3.9	S. Poser (1994)
Hesse (south)	49–50°N	1975–1984	3.8	Lauer & Firnhaber (1994)
Poland				
Szczecin	54°N	1980–1992	2.2	Potemkowski et al. (1994)
Canada				
Barrhead County, Alberta	54°N	1950–1989	3.6	Warren & Warren (1992)
Westlock County, Alberta	54°N	1950–1989	4.0	Warren & Warren (1993)
Saskatoon, Saskatchewan	52°N	1980–1989	9.2	Hader (1999)
Newfoundland	52°N	1960–1982	2.2	Pryse-Phillips (1986)
Winnipeg, Manitoba	50°N	1940–1959	1.5	Stazio et al. (1964)
London, Ontario	43°N	1984	3.4	Hader, Elliot & Ebers (1988)
Netherlands				
Groningen	53°N	1981–1990	3.3	Minderhoud & Zwanniken (1994)
France				
Dijon	47°N	1993–1997	6.1	Moreau et al. (2000)
Hungary				
Fejer	47°N	1972–1991	3.2	Guseo, Jofeju & Kocsis (1994)
Baranya	46°N	1974–1982	0.8	Prange et al. (1986)
Croatia				
Gorski Kotar	45°N	1964–1983	5.9	Sepcic et al. (1989)
Slovenia	45–47°N	1975–1992	2.9	Koncan-Vracko (1994)
Italy				
Aosta	46°N	1976–1985	2.4	Sironi et al. (1991)
Ferrara	45°N	1970–1979	2.2	Granieri et al. (1985)

Table 3. *Continued*

Country and/or region	Latitude	Period	Incidence per 100 000 pop.	References
Sardinia (NW)	41°N	1972–1991	4.6	Rosati et al. (1996)
Tempio	41°N	1977–1985	5.1	Rosati et al. (1991)
Sassari	41°N	1965–1985	3.4	Rosati et al. (1988)
Barbagia	40°N	1971–1980	3.1	Granieri et al. (1983)
Alghero	40°N	1971–1980	7.5	Rosati et al. (1987)
United States				
Rochester, MN	44°N	1905–1984	4.8	Wynn et al. (1990)
Olmstead County, MN	44°N	1905–1984	4.0	Wynn et al. (1990)
Boston, MA	42°N	1954	2.6	Kurland & Westlund (1954)
New Orleans, LA	30°N	1940–1959	0.4	Stazio, Paddison & Kurland (1967)
Spain				
Gijon	43°N	1979–1991	2.1	Uria et al. (1994)
Calatayud	41°N	1980–1989	2.6	Pina et al. (1998)
Alcoi	39°N	1986–1992	3.0	Matias-Guiu et al. (1994)
Greece				
Macedonia and Thrace	40°N	1970–1984	1.8	Milonas, Tsounis & Logothetis (1990)
South Africa (native-born)	30°S	1960	0.4	Dean (1967)
Australia				
Perth, WA	32°S	1950–1981	1.2	Hammond et al. (1988a)
Newcastle, NSW	33°S	1950–1981	2.9	Hammond et al. (1988a)
Hobart, Tas.	43°S	1950–1981	1.7	Hammond et al. (1988a)
New Zealand				
Wellington	41°S	1971	1.9	Hornabrook (1971)

[a] Country names used in this table are those that are valid at the time of publication of this book.

Several surveys have been published of migration from high-risk to low-risk geographical regions, including migration from Europe to Israel, to parts of Africa, and to low-risk areas of Australia. The first study of immigrants, conducted in Israel by Alter, Leibowitz & Speer (1966), observed a lower prevalence of MS among immigrants from northern Europe than would be expected from northern European prevalence rates. Later, Dean & Kurtzke (1971) demonstrated that prevalence rates among immigrants to South Africa from high-risk and medium-risk areas were 48 and 15 per 100 000, respectively, while the rate among native-born residents was 6 per 100 000. Immigrants to the low-risk western part of Australia from high-risk areas had a rate of 31 per 100 000, compared with a rate of 10 among native-born residents; a similar pattern was observed among immigrants to other parts of Australia (Hammond et al., 1988b; Hammond, English & McLeod, 2000). Studies of migration within Australia (Hammond et al., 1988b) and the USA (Kurtzke, Beebe & Norman, 1979) have produced similar findings. For example, Kurtzke, Beebe & Norman (1979) found that armed forces veterans who were born in the northern USA but enlisted in the south had a consistently lower risk than those who were both born and enlisted in the north.

Studies both between and within countries invariably show that immigrants from high-risk to low-risk areas have a higher rate than that in their new homeland, but often somewhat lower than that in their place of origin. If this observation were based only on prevalence data, it might simply reflect the fact that sick and disabled people are less likely to move, rather than less frequent exposure to a risk factor or more frequent exposure to a protective factor in the new place of residence. However, data for the USA are based primarily on incidence and document the same decline in risk as found in prevalence studies.

There are fewer studies of immigrants from low-risk to high-risk areas, but most findings indicate that immigrants retain the same risk as in their countries of origin. This may be because they carry some protective factor with them, but these studies frequently involve non-white immigrants in whom the disease is known to be rare and who may be genetically resistant. Dean et al. (1976) found no increased risk of MS among immigrants to London, England, from low-prevalence areas such as India, Pakistan, and the West Indies, except in the case of mixed-race individuals from the Indian subcontinent who had a British parent. A follow-up study (Dean et al., 1977) shows that, among West Indian immigrants to the United Kingdom, the MS risk is one-eighth that of native-born residents. Kurtzke (1993) has suggested not only that susceptibility is an issue, but also that some of the immigrants in such studies may not have been resident long enough to be exposed to an environmental risk factor or to manifest clinical onset. Within the USA, Detels et al. (1978) found no increased risk among southerners living in Seattle, Washington, although the numbers were very small. Conversely, Kurtzke, Beebe & Norman (1979) reported a consistent increase in MS risk among American armed forces veterans who moved north between birth and enlistment compared with those who remained in the south. Studies from France (Kurtzke & Bui, 1980) and the Netherlands (Dassel, 1972) suggest that the incidence of MS in immigrants from Viet Nam and the Caribbean, respectively, may be higher than in their place of origin. In the French study, however, this conclusion was based on only a few cases, among whom three half-French half-Vietnamese boys reported in Paris should perhaps be disregarded because of their mixed parentage. More recently Kurtzke, Delasnerie-Laupretre & Wallin (1998) studied immigrants from French North Africa to France between 1923 and 1986. Of these 86% were of European origin and the rest were Arab or Berber. In 219 of the 246 cases of MS identified, onset of the disease had occurred *after* migration to France.

There are also a few studies of prevalence rates among the children of immigrants. Elian, Nightingale & Dean (1990) reported that the MS prevalence rate among the British-born children of immigrants from India, Pakistan, and parts of Africa and the West Indies were very much higher than that recorded for their parents and approximately equal to the expected rate for London, England. Biton & Abramsky (1986) have reported that children born to northern European immigrants in Israel have a lower prevalence than would be expected from northern European rates, which suggests that a risk factor may be less common or that the environment in Israel may have some protective effect. On the other hand, there is some debate over prevalence among children born to African and Asian immigrants. Leibowitz, Kahana & Alter (1969) reported a similar rate to that among children of northern European immigrants, whereas the prevalence of MS among their parents had been lower than that among northern European-born parents. If this were indeed the case, it would suggest that the risk to children of African and Asian immigrants was higher than expected, perhaps implying greater exposure to some detrimental factor. However, the observation that there was no difference between these groups of children was apparently based on rates that had been standardized on age and sex to the USA population. C.M. Poser (1994) objects to the use of the very different and heterogeneous population of the USA to adjust Israeli rates, and maintains that a comparison of the children's crude rates is more appropriate. This shows that the difference noted among immigrants persists in their children, implying that the rates among African and Asian children have not risen.

Migration studies have provided information not only on risk changes but also on the age of MS acquisition. In general, research shows that individuals migrating from high-frequency to low-frequency countries carry with them the risk of their country of origin, provided that they migrate after puberty. Conversely, those who move before puberty tend to acquire the lower risk of their country of destination. Europeans migrating to Israel or South Africa before age 15 apparently experience a greater reduction in risk than those who migrate at a later age. Dean & Kurtzke (1971), for example, reported a study of 114 northern European immigrants with MS who were resident in South Africa by 1960, most of whom had migrated after age 15. Among individuals older than 15 at migration, rates were 66/100 000 for immigrants from the United Kingdom and 81/100 000 for all northern Europeans. For those who had migrated between birth and 14 years of age, the rate in both groups was 13/100 000. The inference is that the older immigrants had acquired MS by the time they left their high-risk homelands, while younger immigrants probably acquired the disease after migration to South Africa. A similar pattern was found in a study of American armed forces veterans (Kurtzke, Beebe & Norman, 1979), in which migrating southwards before induction reduced the risk of MS but moving after induction (typically at age 19) had no effect.

Lower rates among those who migrate at a younger age would indicate either the rarity of a geographical risk factor for MS, or the existence of some protective factor, in low-risk areas. The rate among older immigrants, which is intermediate between that in country of origin and that in the new homeland, may also indicate the presence of a protective factor against clinical manifestation of the disease. Recently, however, Hammond, English & McLeod (2000) reported that the prevalence of MS among British and Irish individuals migrating to Australia before the age of 15 was not significantly different from that among people who migrated at or after age 15. On the basis of this observation they raised the possibility that the risk from environmental factors operates over many years and not just in childhood and early adolescence.

Overall, there is consistent evidence that migration from high-risk to low-risk areas in early life is associated with a reduced risk of MS. Likewise, migration from low-risk to high-risk areas probably increases risk although the evidence here is less striking. Since many of the studies of movement from high-risk to low-risk areas essentially control for race or ethnicity, their results implicate either an environmental risk factor, which increases with distance from the Equator, or a protective factor with reciprocal distribution. However, migration studies have not directly attempted to identify such factors.

3.2.4 Geographical clusters

In addition to the general relationship between prevalence and latitude, a number of studies have documented geographical clusters of patients with MS, which may provide valuable clues to disease etiology. Such clusters have received considerable attention from researchers and, since they suggest a harmful shared experience, are often interpreted as evidence of the existence of environmental risk factors.

Prevalence surveys conducted in Europe, for example, have indicated different rates within Denmark, Finland, Norway, northern Scotland, Sweden, and Switzerland. In each of these countries, areas of high prevalence tend to be contiguous, with rates in the areas of highest and lowest prevalence differing by a factor of six or more. By reviewing available mortality and prevalence statistics, Kurtzke (1974) showed an uneven distribution of MS in Scandinavia. A high-risk area spanned southern Norway, extending across southern Sweden to western parts of Finland; there was also a smaller high-risk area within Denmark, located in Funen and Jutland. Scandinavia covers a north–south latitude range from 55° to 70°N, but the north–south MS gradient observed elsewhere was not evident. In fact, the gradient seemed to be reversed, with lower rates in the northern part of Scandinavia. Koch-Henriksen (1995) has confirmed the persistence of this pattern. However, the excess cases within this zone—while statistically significant—may not be biologically significant. Case-ascertainment may be more thorough in densely populated areas, and these areas may also attract MS patients from remote regions who require special services. Nevertheless, Kurtzke (1993) has argued that the six-fold differences are too great to have no biological significance and supported the idea of an environmental MS risk factor.

Many smaller "cluster" foci have been reported throughout the world. Such clusters are often detected in small towns rather than large centres because the patients are more conspicuous and more likely to be exposed to a circumscribed set of possible environmental risk factors. Some of these clusters have not been sustained when tested statistically; others have lost cases when subjected to scrutiny—because of misdiagnosis, for example. Still others, such as that reported in Överkalix, Sweden (Binzer et al., 1994), were the result of familial aggregation.

A number of apparently remarkable clusters consisted of people living close together who experienced onset of symptoms at about the same time but who had grown up elsewhere, or of people born and raised in different areas who happened to manifest the disease while engaged in the same occupation. One of the most famous examples of the latter was that of four of the seven scientists studying swayback in sheep in Scotland who subsequently exhibited symptoms of MS (Campbell et al., 1947). Another interesting cluster consisted of 20 cases reported in Los Alamos County, New Mexico (Hoffman et al., 1981): of the 13 patients in whom onset of symptoms occurred during residence in Los Alamos, nine had migrated to the county after age 15. Many of the patients were employed on the development of the atomic bomb during the Second World War. In a more recently reported cluster in New York state, 20 individuals working in a plant that used zinc as a primary metal developed MS symptoms over a 20-year period—a higher rate than would be expected by chance (Schiffer et al., 1994). If, as most migrant studies indicate, an environmental agent related to acquisition operates before the age of 15 years, such studies can only provide clues to agents that precipitate MS symptoms.

Some recognized clusters have consisted of people who grew up together in the same environment. For example, eight of 11 people assessed as having MS in Henribourg, Saskatchewan, were women who attended the same small school, and seven of them had definitely consumed water from the village common well (Hader, Irvine & Schiefer, 1990). In another instance, eight of 14 patients had lived in close proximity along the main street of a small Massachusetts community about 20 years before the onset of clinical symptoms and during a time when the water supply was contaminated (Eastman, Sheridan & Poskanzer, 1973). Of a cluster of 22 patients with MS in Key West, Florida, 10 had been living in the county before age 15 and seven were nurses (Helmick et al., 1989). One of the significant risk factors was visits to a local military base, which the researchers considered to be a point of similarity to temporal epidemics reported in the Faeroe Islands and Iceland after military occupation during the Second World War. Similar clusters have been reported from Mossyrock, WA, USA (Koch et al., 1974) and Nova Scotia, Canada (Murray, 1976).

One of the obvious difficulties involved in identifying risk factors based on such studies is that the environment may have changed radically by the time the cluster is identified, making past environmental conditions untraceable (Rothman, 1990). Even if this were not a consideration, some researchers (Compston, 1990) have suggested that the majority of clusters that are not reduced by misdiagnosis or because of familial aggregation are probably the result of statistical chance. Because of the localized nature of geographical clusters, the formulation of appropriate denominators is not clear cut. Furthermore, since clusters are identified before speculation about their possible causes, conventional statistical tests are strictly speaking not appropriate. Special statistical tests have been developed to analyse cluster data: the best known include those of Ederer, Myers & Mantel (1964), Knox (1964), Barton, David & Merrington (1965), Mantel (1967), and Breslow & Day (1988). Schottenfeld & Fraumeni (1982) have compared many of these approaches and concluded that no particular method is best. However, more recently Roberson (1990) has criticized the Knox and Mantel methods, since results can be affected by irregular variations in the underlying population distributions. Langmuir (1965) recommended that such tests not be used with clusters, suggesting that clusters should simply be explored for possibly interesting clues to etiology.

A variety of environmental factors including infections, water quality, and occupational exposures could account for geographical clusters. To date, however, no clear causal links have been established.

3.2.5 Temporal clusters or epidemics

A review of MS incidence studies conducted in the same place over time indicates that cyclical fluctuations are not uncommon and are often statistically significant. Large and fleeting excesses in MS frequency, "point epidemics", have not often been reported. However, there has been speculation that two MS epidemics have occurred since the Second World War—in the Faeroe Islands of Denmark and one in Iceland.

In Iceland, the average annual incidence of MS rose from 1.6/100 000 population for the period 1923–1944 to 3.2/100 000 between 1945 and 1954, then dropped again to 1.9/100 000 between 1955 and 1974 (Benedikz et al., 1994). Kurtzke, Guthmundsson & Bergmann (1982) concluded that this incidence pattern met the criteria for a point-source epidemic and was related to the British troop occupation during the Second World War. Their assertion has been contested (Benedikz, Magnusson & Guthmundsson, 1994; Poser CM, 1994) on several grounds. The initial survey in the late 1950s was retrospective, while figures since then have been collected prospectively. Retrospective surveys of MS incidence may produce underestimates because of case-ascertainment deficiencies. In addition, Iceland had no neurology specialists before 1942, and this may have led to both improved recognition of MS and the apparent increase in incidence observed during the next decade. Onset of some of the cases identified between 1945 and 1954 may actually have occurred during the previous period, since Benedikz, Magnusson & Guthmundsson (1994) noted that the interval between clinical onset and diagnosis ranged from 15 to 42 years before 1940, but decreased to 5–7 years thereafter. Finally, the drop in incidence between 1955 and 1974 was followed by an increase to about 3.8/100 000 during the period 1975–1990, representing an overall cyclical pattern rather than a peak followed by a consistent downward trend. Whether the most recent increase is a true increase or the result of more advanced diagnostic techniques is not clear. Regarding a connection between the 1945–1954 peak and troop occupation, Benedikz, Magnusson & Guthmundsson (1994) point out not only that cases of MS had occurred before the arrival of British troops, but that a detailed breakdown of data also shows incidence gradually increasing over the previous 20-year period. In addition, the correspondence between troop locations and where patients lived, either at clinical onset or around age 15 (the suggested age of acquisition), was not particularly remarkable.

The incidence pattern in the Faeroe Islands is more dramatic, with a notable peak and overall consistent downward trend despite cyclical fluctuations following the peak. An intensive retrospective survey by Kurtzke & Hyllested (1979) detected 32 native Faeroese with clinical onset of MS between 1943 and 1973, indicating that MS was relatively common. They were unable to find any patient with clinical onset before the arrival of British troops during the Second World War and concluded that MS was introduced by these troops, resulting in one major and two subsequent minor epidemics. Among patients who were aged 11 years by 1943, 20 represented the first epidemic between 1943 and 1960, nine the second, and three the third. Recently, Kurtzke (1995) reported the discovery of an additional three patients who belong in the third epidemic and seven patients who constitute a fourth. Both Benedikz, Magnusson & Guthmundsson (1994) and C.M. Poser (1994), however, have contested the Faeroese epidemic. Although Kurtzke & Hyllested (1979) reported no cases of MS before the Second World War, Fog & Hyllested (1966) described two death certificates issued between 1930 and 1940 that listed MS as the cause of death. Neither of the two patients concerned had been admitted to hospital with their disease, suggesting that case-ascertainment problems may have contributed to the impression that MS did not exist in the Faeroes prior to 1943.

Acheson (1985) has compared the MS incidence pattern in the Faeroes with data from Orkney and the Shetland Islands collected by Poskanzer et al. (1980a) for the same period. Although the aggregation of cases in the Faeroes between the years 1945 and 1954 was more striking, and the apparent virtual absence of cases before 1943 remarkable, there was a considerable degree of similarity between the incidence patterns in these three island groupings. A formal statistical comparison of the onset distribution of cases showed no statistically significant differences. Unlike the situation in Iceland, Kurtzke & Hyllested (1987) found a positive correlation between the location of British troop encampments and the areas where MS patients lived in the Faeroe Islands. Case–control studies regarding contact have apparently not been conducted, but the researchers have concluded that troops brought a persistent, transmissible infection with them which is responsible for MS.

An examination of reported "outbreaks" of MS among white Afrikaners in South Africa (Rosman, Jacobs & van der Merwe, 1985) and black Kenyans (Adam, 1989) indicates that these were simply the result of an unusual number of patients being diagnosed within a short period of time and probably reflect greater awareness of the disease and improved diagnostic capabilities among local clinicians. An epidemic was also suspected in Macomer, Sardinia (Rosati et al., 1986), where incidence of MS suddenly rose from 0 to 13 cases; however, recalculation of the data, which were based on probable acquisition rather than clinical onset, failed to confirm any outbreak.

Generally speaking, there is no strong evidence to suggest that MS is an epidemic disease. However, several observers remain convinced and in particular suggest that a transmissible disease is implicated: for example, some as yet unidentified persistent infection transmitted from person to person (Kurtzke, 1995) or an animal virus like canine distemper (Cook et al., 1995). Nevertheless, other environmental factors, including toxins introduced into food or water, could be linked to temporal clusters.

3.2.6 Sex-, age-, and race-specific rates

Although MS frequency varies with latitude, its distribution according to sex, age, and race does not. Many clinicians of the early 20th century, including Lord Brain (1930), perceived the risk of MS among males to be equal to or higher than that among females. However, most recent surveys agree that MS is more prevalent among females than males worldwide, with an average female:male ratio of about 1.4:1 (Acheson, 1985). Although some observers have commented that in the early 1900s men would have been more likely than women to receive medical care for MS symptoms, Ajdacic-Gross (1994) has hypothesized that there may have been an actual reversal in the prevalence of MS. His hypothesis is based on an age-cohort analysis using Swiss mortality data from 1901 to 1990. Since the 1.4:1 female:male ratio is based on prevalence rates, it may be influenced by a difference in survival between the sexes; however, median survival for the past few decades seems to be similar in most countries (Kurtzke, 1997).

The female:male mortality ratio varies from a high of 2:1 in New Zealand in the period 1967–1973 (Massey & Schoenberg, 1982) to almost 1:1 in the USA (Chandra et al., 1984). Sex-specific incidence rates are rarely calculated for MS because overall rates are so low. Nevertheless, the sample of studies summarized in Table 4 suggests that incidence is consistently higher in women. This pattern applies until at least age 30, when rates begin to converge (Acheson, 1985). Some researchers have suggested that the difference in incidence between women and men is widening. For example, Kinnunen (1984) noted increases in the female:male ratio in Finland from 1.2:1 to 2.0:1 for Uusimaa and from 1.0:1 to 2.0:1 for Vaasa over the period 1964–1978. Most of this change is accounted for by increased differences in the younger age groups, so that Grønning et al. (1991) have suggested that it is explained by the increased occurrence of the RR form of MS, which is more common in women. However, it may be that improved diagnostic criteria have simply led to earlier diagnosis of the RR form of the disease.

Age-specific incidence and prevalence rates indicate that MS is a major cause of neurological disability among young to middle-aged adults in North America and northern Europe. The risk of first developing MS rises steeply from adolescence, reaching its peak around age 30 and then declining until incidence becomes rare. This pattern is apparent in all areas, regardless of whether the disease is common or uncommon, as illustrated by the representative sample of incidence studies in Fig. 4. Age-specific prevalence rates follow a similar pattern, as shown in Fig. 5, except that the peak rates occur about two decades later, with the highest rates among people in their mid to late 40s. Most studies indicate that the duration of disease varies from 12 to 20 years

Table 4. Female:male ratio for incidence of multiple sclerosis

Country and/or region	Incidence per 100 000 pop.		Ratio F : M	Reference
	Females	**Males**		
Australia				
Perth, WA	1.7	0.6	2.8	Hammond et al. (1988a)
Western Australia	1.5	0.6	2.5	Hammond et al. (1988b)
South Africa (whites)	0.5	0.2	2.5	Dean (1967)
United States				
Rochester, MN	8.5	3.8	2.2	Wynn et al. (1990)
New Orleans, LA	0.6	0.3	2.0	Stazio, Paddison & Kurland (1967)
Boston, MA	4.1	2.3	1.8	Kurland & Westlund (1954)
Finland				
Vaasa	4.2	1.9	2.2	Kinnunen (1984)
Uusimaa	2.5	1.2	2.1	Kinnunen (1984)
New Zealand				
Wellington	2.4	1.3	1.8	Hornabrook (1971)
France				
Dijon	6.1	3.3	1.8	Moreau et al. (2000)
Canada				
Winnipeg, Manitoba	2.7	1.8	1.5	Stazio et al. (1964)
Northern Ireland	2.4	2.0	1.2	Millar (1972)
Denmark	3.7	3.0	1.2	Kurtzke (1968)
Iceland	2.1	2.0	1.1	Benedikz et al. (1994)

(Matthews, 1985), although some have reported durations of up to 35 years (Kurtzke, Dean & Botha, 1970; Percy et al., 1971). In the USA during the 1970s, the highest age-specific, MS-related mortality rates occurred between the ages of 50 and 70. There were peaks at age 60 for white women, 65 for white men, and 55 for non-whites of both sexes (Chandra et al., 1984)—universally earlier than among the general population. Data from Canada indicate peaks at age 60–64 for both women and men in 1980–1984, ages 65–69 and 60–64 for women and men respectively in 1985–1989, and 70–74 versus 60–64 respectively in 1990–1994 (Warren et al., 1999[1]).

All medium- to high-risk areas for MS throughout the world have predominantly white populations. In countries with both white and non-white populations, MS rates are lower among non-whites. For example, the disease is virtually non-existent among Australian Aborigines (Hammond et al., 1988a), New Zealand Maoris (Skegg et al., 1987), and black people in South Africa (Kies, 1989). In the USA, incidence and prevalence rates are twice as high among whites as among African-Americans regardless of latitude; Kurtzke (1993) reports that MS is also less frequent among North American Indians, Latin Americans, and people of the western Pacific region than among whites (Kurtzke, 1993). Likewise, the age-adjusted, average annual MS mortality rates for American whites are considerably higher, at 1.29 for females and

---

[1] *Mortality rates for multiple sclerosis in Canada.* Paper presented at the Regional North American Annual Meeting of the World Federation of Neurology—Research Group of Neuroepidemiology, Toronto.

Fig. 4. Age-specific incidence rates of multiple sclerosis[a]

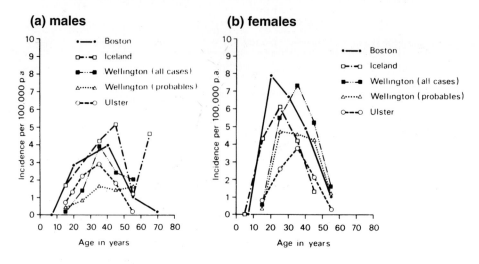

(a) males

(b) females

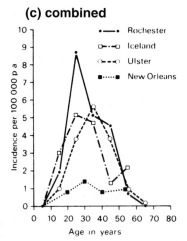

(c) combined

[a] Reproduced from Acheson (1985) with the permission of the publisher, Churchill Livingstone.

0.99 for males, than for non-white females (0.91) and males (0.60) (Chandra et al., 1984).

Like the geographical distribution of MS, distribution of the disease by sex, age, and race or ethnicity has been studied for clues to etiology. No particular underlying risk factors associated with any of these features have been identified.

Fig. 5. Age-specific prevalence rates of multiple sclerosis for various locations[a]

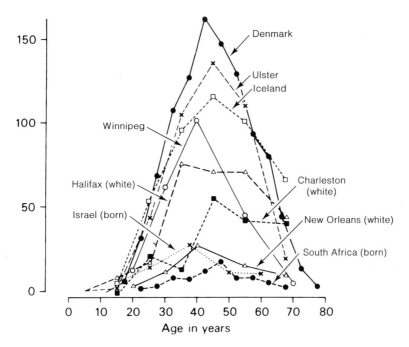

[a] Reproduced from Acheson (1985) with the permission of the publisher, Churchill Livingstone.

3.3 Environmental risk factors

The worldwide distribution of MS can be only an indirect reflection of its cause, implicating some environmental factor that varies with latitude, and can be interpreted in at least three different ways in the search for clues to a specific etiology. First, an environmental risk factor may be more common in temperate than tropical climates. Second, such a factor may be more common in tropical climates where it is acquired at an earlier age and consequently has less impact. Third, this factor may be equally common in all regions, but the chance of its acquisition or of the manifestation of symptoms is either increased by some enhancing factor present in temperate climates or reduced by a protective factor present in tropical areas.

Whatever risk factors are considered they should have some underlying biological plausibility. At present, the most widely held theory is that MS is an autoimmune disease triggered by an as-yet unidentified virus, although other possible triggering agents such as toxins have been considered. Both descriptive and analytical studies have been used to look for associations between environmental factors that may vary with latitude and that either cause the disease directly or influence exposure or reaction to a causal factor.

Descriptive studies, which attempt to correlate the prevalence of MS with the distribution of potential risk factors, have certain methodological limitations. They are usually based on prevalence data so that correlations may not be biologically relevant. In addition, since they are based on aggregate data and do not test hypotheses on individuals, their results are subject to "ecological fallacy": that is, although the prevalence of a suspected risk factor may be high where prevalence is high, individuals within that population who have MS may not necessarily have been exposed to the factor more often than individuals without the disease.

Most analytical studies of MS risk factors are retrospective (or case–control), since low incidence has precluded the prospective approach. Although case–control studies test hypothesis with individuals, they are also subject to some methodological limitations. Very few of the studies conducted to date differentiate between factors that might influence acquisition of the disease and those that would trigger the appearance of clinical symptoms. In other words, they do not differentiate between factors that operate before the age of 15, when acquisition is thought to occur, and those that operate around the time of onset or possibly relapse. The low frequency of the disease often means that numbers of study subjects are small and statistical power is low. In addition, the diagnostic criteria used may make it more difficult to detect differences between cases and controls. Criteria that allow for the inclusion of "possible" cases of MS may result in a significant number of misclassified cases, thus reducing the size of differences observed on suspected risk factors. Using more rigorous criteria, however, may mean that several years elapse between the time when patients first experience symptoms and their classification as "definite"—a delay that may affect patients' recall of events. Since study participants are often interviewed many years after onset (which peaks around age 30), both cases and controls may have inaccurate memories of events or experiences, and cases may be biased if they believe some factor is associated with the disease.

Matching of cases and controls on possibly confounding factors—for example, age, sex, residence before onset, and race or ethnicity—is also important to increase the chance of finding differences on environmental risk factors; the extent of matching varies in analytical studies.

Despite the limitations of both descriptive and analytical approaches, an enormous number of studies of environmental risk factors that might be associated with latitude have been published. These have focused on, among other things, climate and solar radiation, infections and living conditions, and diet and trace elements, but have reached no firm conclusions about the relevance of any of these factors.

3.3.1 Climate and solar radiation

The most obvious environmental factor that varies with latitude is climate. Certain climatic features have been observed to influence immune functions (Afoke et al., 1993), which might be one biological explanation for any relationship between climate and the occurrence of MS. Climate also indirectly influences frequency of exposure to certain viruses, such as those responsible for the respiratory tract infections that are more common in winter and in cold, damp climates (Graham, 1990). It can equally well be argued, however, that warm climates tend to inhibit the spread of respiratory and other infections because of better ventilation, outdoor living, and the sterilizing effect of sunlight. The types and quantities of food produced also vary considerably with climate and this too may influence exposure to some etiological factor.

Consistent with its relationship to latitude, MS is more prevalent in temperate than tropical climates. However, factors other than temperature define climate, and a variety of subclimates exist within both temperate and tropical zones. Lauer (1995) reviewed descriptive studies in several countries including Australia and New Zealand (Miller et al., 1990), Bulgaria (Kalafatova, 1987), Czechoslovakia (Cernacek et al., 1971), France (Alpérovitch & Bouvier, 1982), Turkey (Mutlu, 1960), the USA (Acheson, Bachrach & Wright, 1960), and various other European countries and countries of the former Soviet Union. He concluded that the only highly consistent ecological association that can be established is that between MS frequency and "low" temperature. He noted equivocal correlations with sunshine and also with humidity or precipitation, for which a better fit was obtained when only winter conditions in Australia, France, and the USA were considered.

Similarly, analytical studies have found no differences between MS patients and controls regarding the climates to which they have been exposed. A survey of United States armed forces veterans (Norman, Cook & Dowling, 1983) compared 5305 MS patients with age- and sex-matched controls. The survey concentrated on latitude and on a variety of factors used in the classification of climate, including: mean annual freeze-free period; annual solar radiation; mean annual hours of sunshine; mean annual days with temperature >32°C; mean annual days with temperature <0°C; mean July relative humidity; mean annual pan evaporation; mean annual days of rainfall; and mean annual days forecasted to have air pollution. Individually, each of these factors was highly significant for MS risk. When adjusted for latitude, however, none was found to affect the risk of MS. On the other hand, the relationship with latitude remained significant when adjusted for each of the other variables. The effects of several composite climatic variables (for example, cold and rain) were also examined but no differences were found between cases and controls. Unfortunately no index of winter sunshine, a factor that correlates closely with latitude and has been associated with MS in descriptive studies in Australia, France, and the USA, was included. Despite the possibility that patients are more likely to come from areas with fewer hours of winter sunshine, no difference in frequency of outdoor occupations has been observed between cases and controls (Leibowitz & Alter, 1973; Warren et al., 1982), and no differences in exposure to winter sunshine through recreation have been observed (Warren et al., 1982).

In general, both descriptive and analytical studies suggest that the correlation between latitude and MS prevalence must be explained by other than conventional meteorological variables. Lauer (1995) has suggested the possible value of investigating either solar or terrestrial radiation because of its possible impact on immune function. Barlow (1960) found a correlation between MS mortality rate and cosmic ray intensity, using geomagnetic latitude as a proxy measure, both worldwide and within certain countries such as Australia, Italy, and the USA. Using more recent prevalence data, Resch (1994) confirmed Barlow's findings at the global level and also within the northernmost parts of Europe. Lauer (1995) recommends that terrestrial radiation from radon decay, which is high in mountainous areas (Kreienbrock et al., 1993), should also be explored since several studies have observed excess MS rates in elevated regions (Cernacek et al., 1971; Norman, Cook & Dowling, 1983; Lauer, 1995).

3.3.2 Infections and living conditions

Certain infections, including respiratory tract infections, tend to vary with latitude. Several ubiquitous human viruses have been considered as possible causative agents for MS because they trigger CNS demyelination. Since MS is quite rare, it is difficult to understand how a common infection might be involved in its etiology. MS might be an uncommon complication of some minor infection that is clinically indistinguishable from many others, like the common cold and influenza, so that its role as a precursor is missed. Conversely, an easily recognizable virus such as the measles virus might cause MS, but MS would be such an unusual consequence, with symptoms occurring after a long latency period, that the association would be overlooked.

A number of animal viruses can also produce CNS demyelinating disease with exacerbations and remissions as well as progression. Some researchers have therefore suggested that MS may even result from an infection normally hosted by animals, but occasionally infecting humans when it may or may not be diagnosed. In any case, an additional susceptibility factor (possibly environmental and related to latitude) would have to influence which individuals exposed to an infectious agent developed MS. For example, certain living conditions in tropical climates, such as poverty, crowding, and poor sanitation, promote the early occurrence of infections when they may have less impact, as is the case for poliomyelitis (Poskanzer, Schapira & Miller, 1963b).

Several human viruses, including the measles virus, the coronavirus 229E, parvovirus B19, hepatitis B virus, and the Epstein–Barr virus (human (gamma) herpesvirus 4), have been considered as possible causes of MS. Measles has received the most attention despite the fact that descriptive studies do not indicate any correlation between the occurrence of measles virus infections and the worldwide distribution of MS, including the north–south gradient and geographical clusters (Cook et al., 1995). By contrast, there is considerable evidence that the prevalence of respiratory infections, such as group A β-haemolytic streptococcal infections, increase with distance from the Equator.

Analytical studies comparing the frequency of various infections in MS patients and in controls have shown an increased frequency of a number of infections in MS patients, but no specific infection has been consistently implicated (Acheson, 1985). Nevertheless, reported differences do lean towards excess occurrence in MS patients, possible indicating a generally greater susceptibility to infection. Warren et al. (1985a) compared optic neuritis patients who developed MS with those who did not, and found that the MS patients experienced a greater number of childhood infections and more frequent colds, streptococcal infections, herpes labialis, and tonsillitis. Infections have also been associated with MS relapses in other studies (Sibley, Bamford & Clark, 1985; Gay, Dick & Upton, 1986). In several case–control studies that have considered childhood infectious diseases, measles has been found to occur later in MS patients (Alter & Cendrowski, 1976; Poskanzer et al., 1980b; Schonberger et al., 1981; Haile et al., 1982; Sullivan, Visscher & Detels, 1984; Alter et al., 1986; Alvord et al., 1987; Grønning et al., 1993); in addition, measles does tend to occur at a later age in temperate climates (Fraser, 1975). Nevertheless, there have been documented cases of measles virus infection after the onset of MS, so that measles immunization has clearly failed to prevent MS (Cook et al., 1995). Any role for measles virus in the causation of MS continues to be debatable, as does the involvement of other specific human viruses.

Various animal viruses have also been suggested as a cause of MS, including canine distemper virus and the virus that causes visna in sheep. Initially, descriptive studies looked for associations between MS prevalence and the worldwide distribution of farm animals or household pets. The only positive correlation observed for farm animals is with cattle rather than sheep, and thus tends to discount a role for visna (Malosse & Perron, 1993; Lauer, 1995). There is also no proven correlation between MS and household pets, including dogs (Malosse & Perron, 1993): canine distemper virus occurs in all climates and its occurrence does not follow the same geographical pattern as MS (Acheson, 1985). Nevertheless, some temporal "variations" have been attributed to canine distemper outbreaks. For example, the islands of Sitka, Alaska, had never reported either MS or canine distemper until the 1970s, when five cases of MS occurred in the 5 years following a documented outbreak of canine distemper (Cook & Dowling, 1981). In Newfoundland, Canada, periodic upswings in MS incidence from 1960 onwards reflected local outbreaks of canine distemper with a lag time of 3–5 years (Pryse-Phillips, 1986).

In analytical studies, case–control comparisons have generally supported the findings of descriptive studies regarding farm animals. Although some researchers have observed more frequent exposure to dogs among MS patients than controls (Chan, 1977; Cook & Dowling, 1977; Jotkowitz, 1977; Cook et al., 1978; Flodin et al., 1988; Landtblom et al., 1993), several others have found no significant difference (Poskanzer, Prenney & Sheridan, 1977; Bunnell, Visscher & Detels, 1979; Sylwester & Poser, 1979; Hughes et al., 1980; Read et al., 1982; Warren et al., 1982; Anderson et al., 1984). At least one case–control study has indicated that MS patients are more likely to keep their dogs indoors, especially in cold, damp climates, which would increase exposure to any illness their pets might be carrying (Norman, Cook & Dowling, 1983). In fact, some studies have found that MS patients are more likely to have been exposed to a dog with distemper or a distemper-like illness (Cook, Dowling & Russell 1978; Norman, Cook & Dowling, 1983; Warren et al., 1982), but others have not (Bauer & Wikström, 1978; Hughes et al., 1980; Read et al., 1982). To add to these conflicting results, human infection with the distemper virus had not been recorded by the mid-1990s, so the possible role of CDV in MS remains highly controversial.

Socioeconomic status and several other factors such as housing density and sanitation probably influence the chance of encountering infections—and possibly the age at which infections develop. The worldwide distribution of MS supports the hypothesis of Poskanzer, Schapira & Miller (1963b) that poor sanitation in the less affluent, tropical regions protects against MS because some causal infection occurs at a younger age when it has less impact. The hypothesis may also be supported by the higher MS risk among the more favoured socioeconomic groups, who would probably be subject to later infection, even in temperate climates, as a result of better sanitation and less crowded living conditions. Socioeconomic status (usually defined by occupation or education) has been investigated largely in analytical studies. Two large studies, one from Northumberland, England (Miller et al., 1960), and one covering the entire USA (Beebe et al., 1967), indicated that MS patients tend to be from a higher socioeconomic background. However, the vast majority of studies produce negative results, including surveys from Edmonton (Warren et al., 1982) and Winnipeg, Canada (Stazio, Paddison & Kurland, 1967), Northern Ireland (Allison & Millar, 1954), Israel (Antonovsky et al., 1968), the Orkney and Shetland Islands (Poskanzer et al., 1980b), and Olmsted County, USA (Kranz, 1982).

Descriptive studies have indicated correlations between MS and both good sanitation and low population density in Wales (Swingler & Compston, 1988) and the USA (Lauer, 1994). A study in Mexico (Gonzalez & Sotelo, 1995) also showed an increase in the number of MS patients presenting at the National Institute of Neurology and Neurosurgery over the previous 20 years during which there were improvements in sanitation. However, several researchers have found no differences between sanitation conditions in the homes of patients and controls (Westlund &

Kurland, 1953b; Antonovsky et al., 1968; Cendrowski et al., 1969; Poskanzer et al., 1980b; Warren et al., 1984; Lauer & Firnhaber, 1994). Other researchers have observed that MS patients came from areas of greater population density than controls (Warren et al., 1984), as did optic neuritis patients who went on to develop MS compared with those who did not (Warren et al., 1985a). On the whole, there is little evidence to support the idea that lower socioeconomic status confers any protection against MS.

Although many researchers believe that a virus is involved in the etiology of MS, the evidence is actually quite weak. Analytical studies have not consistently implicated any human or animal virus and no agent has been repeatedly isolated from MS tissues. Viral particles have not been convincingly demonstrated by electron microscopy, and neither antigen nor genome has been consistently observed in MS specimens using advanced molecular techniques. It has been suggested that a variety of different viruses may trigger MS in susceptible individuals and that those viruses do not necessarily persist, which would account for failure to identify a specific viral agent (Batchelor, 1985). The recent identification of the autoimmune myelin basic protein epitope $Pro_{85}VVHFFKNIVTPro_{96}$ for both T cells and B lymphocyte autoantibodies provides new avenues to explore for the specific virus and/or bacterial amino acid sequence of proteins that may trigger MS by a molecular mimicry mechanism (Warren, Catz & Steinman, 1995; Wucherpfenning & Strominger, 1995).

3.3.3 Diet and trace elements

Since the types and quantity of food produced vary with latitude, some dietary factor may contribute to the etiology of MS. Such a factor could be toxic or might protect against occurrence of the disease. If some type of food is indeed involved, its distribution probably varies according to the distribution of MS: a toxic factor would be more common in high-risk areas and a protective factor more common in low-risk areas. The production pattern of some fruits, cereals, and vegetables is similar to the pattern of MS distribution, as is the consumption of both meat and dairy products, implying an underlying etiological factor. Researchers have also suggested that MS may be related to deficiency of a particular vitamin or of an essential trace element, or to the toxic effect of a heavy metal in the soil or drinking-water of high-risk areas. The biological explanation for a relationship between some type of food or trace element and MS would differ somewhat according to the specific factor.

Food antigens, immunostimulating lectins, and plant pathogens might each form the basis of a biological explanation for any relationship between MS and a particular fruit, cereal, or vegetable. Although production of many of these foods varies with latitude, most are so freely marketed throughout the world that they are unlikely to be involved. Two particular cereals, wheat and oats, have received some attention from researchers. From the distribution of wheat, Shatin (1964) hypothesized that gluten might play a role in the etiology of MS, but Lauer (1995) found no correlation between wheat production and MS rates in various countries worldwide. Although Lauer observed a correlation between MS and oat production, providing support for the hypothesis of Palo, Wikström & Kivalo (1973) that oat-sterile dwarf mosaic virus might cause MS, he found no difference between MS patients and controls in terms of oat consumption in a follow-up study. The possible role of other specific cereals, fruits, or vegetables remains largely unexplored. Some diseases have been linked to these foods, however: for example, ingestion or even contact with the fava bean produces haemolytic anaemia in individuals with a hereditary deficiency of the enzyme glucose-6-phosphate dehydrogenase. A similar etiological factor in MS cannot be entirely dismissed.

More attention has been paid to the possible role of meat and dairy product consumption in MS etiology. The biological explanations for any such relationship include the influence of animal fat both on the membrane composition of myelin and inflammatory mediators such as prostaglandins and leukotrienes, and on the possible transmission of an animal virus. MS is rare in tropical countries, where the consumption of meat and dairy products is low, and more common in temperate climates where consumption is high.

Descriptive studies have generally found a correlation between MS rates and meat consumption at the global level (Agranoff & Goldberg, 1974; Alter, Yamoor & Harshe, 1974; Knox, 1977; Nanji & Narod, 1986) and within countries like Norway (Swank et al., 1952) and the USA (Lauer, 1994). An even higher correlation has been observed for dairy products globally (Agranoff & Goldberg, 1974; Knox, 1977; Malosse & Perron, 1993), throughout a number of European countries (Lauer, 1994), and within the USA (Lauer, 1994). Likewise, correlations have been found between dietary fat in general and global MS rates (Esparza, Sasaki & Kesteloot, 1995). However, a convincing majority of analytical studies have found no difference in meat consumption in general between MS patients and controls (Antonovsky et al., 1968; Cendrowski et al., 1969; Warren et al., 1982; Warren et al., 1984; Berr et al., 1989; Murrell and Matthews, 1990; Sepcic et al., 1993), and the findings regarding dairy product consumption have been inconsistent.

In some studies more directly focused on biological mechanisms, an excess intake of animal fat, and especially butter, has been found in MS patients (Murrell & Matthews, 1990; Sepcic et al., 1993; Granieri & Tola, 1994; Lauer & Firnhaber, 1994; Wender & Kazmierski, 1994). Several researchers have also linked the consumption of potentially contaminated meat or milk to MS, including an excess intake of animal brain (Poskanzer et al., 1980b), raw meat (Murrell & Matthews, 1990), uninspected meat/game (Warren et al., 1984), and unpasteurized milk (Murrell & Matthews, 1990; Sepcic et al., 1993). Lauer (1995) has proposed the alternative explanation that meat preparation may be a factor, specifically through a possible immunological hapten role for nitrophenol compounds found in smoked meat.

Descriptive studies have found a correlation between MS rates and smoke-curing methods in various geographical regions, including both France and Switzerland (Lauer, 1989) as well as in eastern Mediterranean areas (Lauer, 1991). This hypothesis is also compatible with the MS "epidemic" in the Faeroe Islands, which peaked at a time when peat-smoking of meat was transitorily common (Lauer, 1989) and declined after this practice ended abruptly in the 1950s (Joensen, 1982). Lauer (1995) has completed a preliminary case–control analysis that indicates an excess risk of benign MS associated with "saltpetre/nitrite use", especially in combination with purchased coniferous timber for smoking. Sepcic et al. (1993) have also observed an elevated risk of MS associated with the consumption of smoked pork. Despite the various plausible mechanisms offered, no factor associated with meat or dairy product consumption has been clearly implicated in the etiology of MS.

Several researchers have hypothesized that a vitamin deficiency might be associated with MS, particularly vitamin D deficiency (Goldberg, 1974; Craelius, 1978; Cantorna, 2000). Certain fish, which are an excellent source of vitamin D, are widely consumed in a number of countries where MS prevalence is low, including Japan (despite a climate classified as temperate) and Greenland. Swank et al. (1952) observed that MS is less common in the coastal fishing communities of Norway than in the inland farming areas. Moreover, vitamin D is synthesized in the skin under the influence of ultraviolet light, which could explain the inverse relationship between winter sunshine and MS. Demyelinated nerve fibres are apparently sensitive to changes in the concentration of calcium ions, which would be one possible biological explanation for the role of vitamin D deficiency. Alternatively, vitamin D may affect the immune system: recent studies indicate that deficiency of vitamin D increases the severity of experimental autoimmune encephalomyelitis, a mouse model of MS (Cantorna, 2000).

Some researchers have suggested that vitamin A deficiency may be involved since it could contribute to a deficiency of system antioxidants that inhibit leukotriene synthesis (Hutter, 1993). Butcher (1992) has also postulated that a problem with calcium metabolism may be etiologically important, on the basis of epidemiological evidence that MS patients report high childhood milk intake followed by a large or sudden reduction during the adolescent growth spurt. However, no analytical study has yet indicated that MS patients are deficient in any vitamin or its metabolites (Acheson, 1985).

It has been suggested by other researchers that MS may be related to the deficiency of an essential trace element, or to the toxic effect of a heavy metal, such as lead, in soil or drinking-water. In general, the geographical distribution of MS is too wide to suggest an association with any particular geological formation, geochemical factor, or soil type except the possibility of peat surface. Peat formation occurs only at high latitudes, and Warren, Delavault & Cross (1967) have suggested that concentrations of heavy metals in acid water supplies derived from peaty soils may be involved in the etiology of MS. The risk of MS does tend to be high in regions characterized by a large proportion of peat surface, including Finland, Ireland, and Scotland. Local associations have also been observed in Northern Ireland (Millar, 1966), north-western Poland (Potemkowski et al., 1994), and parts of the former Soviet Union (Boiko, 1994). From an analysis of 26 countries, Lauer (1995) reported a threefold greater MS risk in countries where peat production is above the median compared with those below the median, although there was no significant correlation when each country's actual peat production was used rather than the above/below median dichotomy. Moreover, water supplies in areas where MS rates are high are not always acid.

Descriptive studies have found no convincing or consistent correlations between MS prevalence and various minerals in drinking-water, including lead, chromium, and selenium (Lauer, 1995). In fact, Lauer & Firnhaber (1992) found a negative correlation between MS mortality and lead in the drinking-water of 35 counties in the German state of Baden-Württemberg. For the MS cluster in Henribourg, Saskatchewan, an extensive study of drinking-water also found a low lead concentration (Irvine, Schieter & Hader, 1989). Among analytical studies, the survey of USA armed forces veterans (Norman, Cook & Dowling, 1983) found no difference, after latitude was taken into account, between patients and controls on the "concentration of dissolved minerals" in the groundwater of areas where they had lived. No biologically plausible explanation has yet been advanced for a relationship between lead or any other mineral and MS.

There is currently less support for the involvement of some dietary factor or trace element in the etiology of MS than there is for the involvement of a viral infection. Nevertheless, researchers continue to study this possibility; since dietary factors and trace elements have been linked to a variety of other diseases, it cannot be ruled out.

3.3.4 Is there an environmental risk factor for multiple sclerosis?

Although the evidence remains elusive, few researchers would argue against the role of an environmental risk factor in MS etiology. The worldwide distribution of MS, migration studies, and geographical and temporal clusters all support the theory that some exogenous variable (probably related to latitude) is necessary for acquisition of the disease. An additional exogenous factor may enhance acquisition or clinical manifestation in regions where the disease is common or offer protection where the disease is rare. However, partly because epidemiological studies have failed to identify any clear-cut environmental risk factor, more attention has recently focused on the possible contribution of genetic susceptibility.

3.4 Genetic susceptibility

The possible etiological role of genetic factors in MS was first suggested almost 90 years ago by Eichhorst (1913), who noticed a familial predisposition to the disease. In 1922 Davenport introduced the idea of racial or ethnic susceptibility when he suggested that the high prevalence of MS among American armed forces veterans of the First World War living in the Great Lakes area might be explained by the high proportion of Scandinavian residents. Subsequent research on MS prevalence in various racial or ethnic groups, and extensive surveys of familial MS that included twins and adopted children, have substantiated the idea of a genetic factor. The first direct evidence came in the early 1970s with the discovery of an association between MS and the alleles of the human leukocyte antigen (HLA) system. Since the major histocompatibility complex (MHC) has been found to encode immune response genes in mice, it is suggested that MS develops in individuals because they inherit an allele that renders them vulnerable to a particular immunological stimulus (possibly viral) leading to a chain of events resulting in myelin injury. An exogenous stimulus is allowed for because the same epidemiological studies that support a genetic contribution also indicate an environmental determinant (Compston, 1999).

3.4.1 Race and ethnicity

Initially, researchers linked the worldwide distribution of MS to some environmental factor that varied with latitude, becoming more common as distance from the Equator increased. Observed lower MS rates among non-whites, who typically inhabit tropical climates, than among whites, who inhabit temperate climates, were attributed to less frequent exposure to an environmental factor, although the possibility of genetic resistance was acknowledged. However, as exceptions to the latitude rule accumulated, some researchers began to suggest that the geographical distribution of MS might be largely explained by the genetic make-up of local inhabitants rather than by uneven global distribution of an environmental cause. Most studies that have addressed this issue are descriptive in nature, and consequently subject to ecological fallacy.

One of the earliest notable exceptions to the "latitude rule" was Japan, where MS prevalence is uniformly low despite the country's northern latitude and temperate climate. Several prevalence studies have been conducted throughout Japan (from 26° to 44°N latitude). Rates range from 0.8/100 000 in Miyazaki to 4.0/100 000 in Morioka, but the 95% CIs generally overlap so that there is no particular variation by geography (Poser CM, 1994). MS rates have not increased since the 1950s, although there have been some dramatic environmental changes. These observations indicate that the low Japanese rate may be explained by genetic resistance; however, cultural patterns such as relatively low consumption of animal fats might also play a role. Since Japan has a relatively homogeneous non-caucasian population, the effect of race is difficult to assess.

In countries with a mix of white and non-white populations, non-whites seem more resistant to MS. Rates of MS among Japanese born in the states of Hawaii (Alter et al., 1971; Shibasaki, Okihiro & Kuroiwa, 1978), California, and Washington (Detels et al., 1977) are higher than rates among Japanese living in Japan (Kuroiwa, Shibasaki & Ikeda, 1983), but still relatively low compared with whites living in those states. Similarly, MS occurs more frequently in African-Americans than in black Africans but less frequently than in the white American population (Kurtzke, Beebe & Norman, 1979). MS rates are also lower among Chinese, Filipinos, and Latin Americans than among whites in the USA (Kurtzke, Beebe & Norman, 1979). MS has never been reported in pure Inuits or North American Indians living in Canada, in Australian Aborigines, or in New Zealand Maoris.

It may be that these groups are genetically resistant or that some aspect of their culture protects against MS. The intermediate MS rates of groups like African-Americans may be the result of racial intermingling: the fact that MS prevalence is higher among African Americans living in the northern states (where there is purported to be more intermingling) than in the southern states is sometimes used to argue this point. However, the intermediate rates of both Japanese-Americans and African-Americans may also indicate that the USA environment is characterized by a factor that enhances the risk of MS acquisition or onset. This factor may increase with distance from the Equator, which provides an alternative explanation for the north–south gradient among African-Americans.

Not only do non-whites have lower MS rates than whites in mixed-race countries, but there are also numerous examples of differing rates among white subgroups as well as among non-white subgroups living within the same country. This holds true whether the country is one of generally high risk or generally low risk. For example: Hutterites in Canada and the northern USA have low MS rates compared with other white North Americans (Hader, 1989[1]); MS has never been recorded in Scandinavian Lapps (Koch-Henriksen, 1995); and MS occurs more frequently among English-speaking whites than among Afrikaners in South Africa (Poser CM, 1994). Among non-white subgroups, MS occurs more frequently in African-Americans than in Japanese-Americans (Kurtzke, Beebe & Norman, 1979), and in Parsees than in Hindus living in either Bombay or Poona, India (Wadia & Bhatia, 1990).

Various other examples of this phenomenon are found throughout the world. In the United Kingdom, for instance, MS is more frequent in the white population of north-eastern Scotland (Grampian region), the Orkneys, and the Shetland Islands than in western Scotland or most parts of England, Wales, and Northern Ireland (Robertson & Compston, 1995). In Uzbekistan, ethnic Russians have significantly higher

---

[1] *MS in Canadian Indians and Hutterites.* Paper presented at a Workshop on Genes and Susceptibility to Multiple Sclerosis, Cambridge University.

prevalence rates than Uzbeks and Bahara Jews (Alaev, 1994). In the German state of Hesse, Turkish workers have a lower prevalence of MS than the general population (Lauer & Firnhaber, 1994), and Hungarian gypsies have a lower rate than native Hungarians (Palffy, 1982; Milanov et al., 1999). Sardinians have a much higher MS rate than mainland Italians, and prevalence rates vary considerably within both mainland Italy and Sicily (Piazza et al., 1988). In Israel, the Ashkenazi Jews have a higher MS rate than the Sephardic Jews (Biton & Abramsky, 1986). Palestinian Arabs living in Kuwait have double the MS rate of Kuwaiti Arabs (Al Din et al., 1991). These and other examples tend to suggest that genetic susceptibility is more important than geography, but some aspect of cultural environment might still explain such variations.

Several researchers have recently suggested that the entire global north–south MS gradient can largely be explained by race or ethnicity, and data largely from the USA have been used to explore this theory. In support of Davenport's 1922 observation, Bulman & Ebers (1992) and Page et al. (1993), analysing data on American armed forces veterans of the Second World War, both found a positive correlation at the state level between MS risk and proportion of residents with Scandinavian ancestry. Apart from the possibility of ecological fallacy, other methodological problems are involved in extrapolating from such descriptive studies like these, such as the fact that MS rates are usually not based on incidence, and questions about the accuracy of population ancestry data reported by local residents. Even if these problems can be overlooked, the correlation between MS prevalence and race or ethnicity does not rule out an environmental risk factor.

Kurtzke (1993) included latitude as a variable in his analysis of the data on American armed forces veterans and found that its contribution to the north–south prevalence gradient in the USA was independent of the ancestry of local residents. Page et al. (1995) correlated MS risk among American veterans with ethnicity derived from surnames and found that risk was more strongly associated with latitude and population ancestry of the state from which servicemen entered service than it was with ethnicity.

While parental ancestry may partially explain the USA gradient, the Australian north–south gradient cannot be explained by either race or ethnicity. Two studies separated by 30 years confirm that the prevalence of MS among whites increases with latitude. Prevalence in Hobart, Tasmania, is twice that in the southern Australian cities of Perth and Newcastle (McLeod, Hammond & Hallpike, 1994), even though the populations of both areas are predominantly descendants of settlers from England, Scotland, and Ireland.

Warren et al. (1996) combined descriptive and analytical methods to examine race or ethnicity as a risk factor for MS in Alberta, Canada. They not only looked for correlations between population ancestry data and MS prevalence rates in the 19 census divisions of the province, but also compared the self-reported parental ancestry of 276 MS patients attending the University of Alberta MS Clinic with the ancestry of controls. At the descriptive level, there was a positive correlation between Scandinavian ancestry and MS prevalence for men only and negative correlations with aboriginal ancestry for both men and women. There were no patients with aboriginal ancestry in the case–control study, which tends to confirm that aboriginal ancestry somehow protects against MS. However, the descriptive-level correlation between Scandinavian ancestry and MS prevalence for men was not confirmed when patients were compared with controls. Besides noting the possibility of inaccurate self-reported ancestry, the researchers also acknowledged the problem of small numbers of both patients and controls reporting single ancestry (both parents from the same background) so that statistical power was quite low. In fact, when comparisons were based on British versus nonspecific European parental ancestry, there was a significant excess MS risk associated with European ancestry for men and a similar trend for women. Larger analytical studies need to be conducted in countries such as Canada and the USA to clarify the impact of specific parental ancestries on MS occurrence, and whether higher prevalence rates at higher latitudes are a reflection of the racial or ethnic backgrounds of residents.

3.4.2 Familial risk studies

Even before researchers began to use prevalence studies to examine racial or ethnic susceptibility, Curtius (1933) observed a familial aggregation of MS cases. Most studies of familial MS have been conducted among whites living in high-risk areas, notably Canada and the United Kingdom. Familial rates are calculated from data on the frequency of MS among the family members of affected individuals (index patients), typically collected using the family history method. Estimates of the percentage of index patients with one or more affected family members have varied from 3.6% (Muller, 1953) to 20% (Sadovnick, Baird & Ward, 1988) and 40.9% (Roberts, Roberts & Poskanzer, 1979). Differences in methodology undoubtedly contribute to these variations. Lower rates are likely to be observed when only first-degree relatives (parents, siblings, and children) of MS index patients are studied and second- and third-degree relatives are excluded. Lower rates may also result from underestimation of affected relatives if only the index patient is interviewed: this individual may be unaware of the existence of other affected relatives or some relatives may have undiagnosed disease. On the other hand, informants may over-report cases of MS on the basis of possible indications of disease among family members. For example, Eldridge et al. (1978) found that 50% of families in which more than one member was reported to have MS had to be rejected because of inaccurate information.

The most accurate studies are probably those that interview multiple informants, and those that employ a neurologist experienced in the differential diagnosis of MS to confirm reported cases among relatives, either through direct assessment or review of clinical/autopsy records. Rates are likely to be higher in studies that include individuals diagnosed with possible MS and isolated ON or that use appropriate laboratory tests, including MRI, to diagnose clinically symptomatic MS. Rates are also likely to be higher when studies incorporate age adjustment. Longitudinal studies clearly indicate that the clinical "affected" status of MS patients' relatives, especially children, tends to rise over time. Affected status should also control for the sex distribution of a particular study group, since MS is characterized by a preponderance of women.

Recurrence risks for affected family members (expressed as the percentage of those at risk who develop MS) have been established in very large series. In most multiplex families (i.e. those in which more than one member has MS), only two relatives are affected. Sadovnick, Baird & Ward (1988) have provided the most detailed breakdown of familial risks, summarized in Table 5. Their observation that the greatest risk is for siblings is consistent with other studies, although it is high at 3.88%; the next highest figure comes from Sutherland (1956) at 1.27%, followed by Schapira, Poskanzer & Miller (1963) at 1.16%, and Allison & Millar (1954) at 1.15%. The Sadovnick, Baird & Ward study also indicates that the risk for parents and children is similar at 2.58% and 2.52% respectively. Although these figures are again high in comparison with other studies, the similarity of risk for parents and offspring has been substantiated by other researchers, including Schapira, Poskanzer & Miller (1963).

There has been some inconsistency in the pattern of risks reported for first-degree familial subgroups. Sadovnick, Baird & Ward (1988) observed that the greatest risks were for daughters of female patients followed by brothers of male patients, while Robertson & Compston (1995) reported the greatest risks for daughters of male patients followed by sisters of female patients. In both studies, however, there was a diminishing risk among second-degree relatives (aunts/uncles) and third-degree relatives (nieces/nephews and cousins), an observation that has also been reported by Roberts & Bates (1982).

Table 5. Familial multiple sclerosis risks[a]

| | Age-adjusted risks | | | |
| | Male index patients | | Female index patients | |
Relationship to index patient	%	n	%	n
Mother	3.84	7/184	3.71	14/383
Father	0.79	1/128	2.00	6/303
Daughter	5.13	2/223	4.96	5/386
Son	0	0/248	0	0/411
Sister	3.46	9/340	5.65	25/608
Brother	4.15	10/326	2.27	10/612
Aunt/uncle	2.68	15/560	1.59	23/1491
Niece/nephew	1.47	3/1000	1.83	7/1789
First cousins	1.53	7/795	2.37	34/2347

[a] As reported by the University of British Columbia Multiple Sclerosis Clinic, Canada (Sadovnick, 1994).

It is immediately clear that the familial risks observed indicate a much greater frequency of MS in relatives of index cases than would be expected among controls, based on the prevalence of MS in the general population. However, this increased risk may be the result of genetic transmission, exposure to a common environment, or both. Researchers have commented that the excess occurrence of MS among second- and third-degree relatives supports the idea of genetic transmission, since common environmental exposures are unlikely (although not impossible if culturally linked, for example). More recently, Gaudet et al. (1995) observed that MS patients are randomly ordered by birth within multiplex sibships where more than one sibling has MS, suggesting that this contradicts the hypothesis that MS occurs in siblings as a result of a common environmental exposure. In addition, Sadovnick et al. (1996) reported a reduction in risk from full siblings to half-siblings (3.5% to 1.2% respectively), interpreting this as supporting the idea that familial aggregation of MS is genetic. However, there is no particular reason to believe that siblings raised together and who are close in age share more of their environment than siblings further removed by birth order, or that half-siblings—who are more likely to be raised apart—are not less likely to be exposed to a contributing environmental risk.

3.4.3 Twins

Studies of twins have provided additional information about MS recurrence risk among siblings. Comparison of concordance rates in monozygotic twins, dizygotic twins, and non-twin siblings is the classic method of exploring the relative etiological importance of genetic versus environmental factors. Monozygotic twins are genetically identical, while dizygotic twins are no more genetically alike than non-twin siblings. However, dizygotic twins may theoretically share a more common environment than non-twin siblings because they are the same age and normally raised in similar circumstances. If a disease is entirely determined by genetics, the concordance rate for monozygotic twins should be 100%. On the other hand, monozygotic concordance rates can be less than 100% for fundamentally genetic disease in which chance environmental factors also play a role. Comparison of concordance rates between dizygotic twins and non-twin siblings measures the influence of non-genetic factors. If there is an important environmental cause, concordance rates should be higher among dizygotic twins on the assumption that they share a more common environment.

Twin studies can be difficult to conduct accurately because of problems with case-ascertainment. Most early twin studies in MS acquired participants through advertising, since there are few patient populations with a large enough number of twins to allow population-based studies. Recruitment of volunteers through public announcements tends to result in an overrepresentation of concordant pairs, probably because they are more motivated to participate in a genetic study than twins of whom only one is affected. Varying estimates of risk for monozygotic and dizygotic

Table 6. *Results from population based twin studies*

Country	Concordance				References
	Monozygotic twins		Dizygotic twins		
	%	n	%	n	
Canada	30.80	8/26	4.70	2/43	Sadovnick et al. (1993)
Denmark	21.05	4/19	3.57	1/28	Heltberg & Holm (1982)
Finland	28.57	2/7	0	0/16	Kinnunen et al. (1988)
France	5.90	1/17	2.70	1/37	French Research Group (1992)
United Kingdom	25.00	11/44	3.30	2/61	Mumford et al. (1992)

twins based on volunteer studies have been attributed to variations in the proportion of concordant twins who may have volunteered.

One measure of ascertainment bias in such studies is the ratio of monozygotic to dizygotic twins in the study sample. Twins occur in approximately one in 80 births, with an expected monozygotic to dizygotic ratio of 1:2. Samples that differ substantially from this ratio should be suspected of bias. The study conducted by Mackay & Myrianthopoulos (1966) comprised considerably more monozygotic pairs than expected, so that their unusually high concordance rate of 20.7% (6/29) for dizygotic twins might be suspect, although the rate of 23.1% (9/39) for monozygotic twins is consistent with more recent population-based studies (see Table 6). Cendrowski et al (1969) reported a typical concordance rate of 26.6% (24/90) for monozygotic twins but an atypically high rate of 12.9% (11/85) for dizygotic twins compared with population-based studies. Bobowick et al. (1978) found the reverse in their study, which had not only a preponderance of monozygotic twins but also small numbers; they reported an unusually high concordance rate for monozygotic twins of 40.0% (2/5) but 0% (0/4) for dizygotic twins. An atypically high rate for both monozygotic twins at 50.0% (6/12) and dizygotic twins at 16.7% (2/12) was reported by Williams et al. (1980).

Several recent twin studies have minimized ascertainment bias by identifying twin pairs from large populations either of MS patients or of twins. As Table 6 shows, four of these studies found a significantly higher clinical concordance rate (about 26%) in monozygotic than in dizygotic twins (about 4%) where any pairs existed. Only the French Research Group (1992) study shows no significant difference between monozygotic and dizygotic pairs. Similar findings from studies in Canada (Sadovnick et al., 1993) and the United Kingdom (Mumford et al., 1992), which used different methods of recruitment, support the validity of these results. Both samples are representative of MS in terms of sex distribution, clinical classification, disease severity, and MRI support. Twins in the Canadian study were recruited from among patients attending university-affiliated MS clinics, which see most of the patients in their local populations, and in the United Kingdom study from neurologists, whereas the French study identified twins from a large cohort of MS patients recruited for other purposes through the media. Nevertheless, patients in the French study are representative of MS patients in general.

Monozygotic twin pairs appear to be overrepresented in the Canadian and British studies but not in the French study. The concordance rates for monozygotic twins in the French study may be underestimates because of sampling bias. The 95% CI for monozygotic twins in the French study (5.9%: 95% CI = 0–17.1%) overlaps with the Canadian study (25.9%: 95% CI = 13–42.5%), as do the CIs for the dizygotic rates in France (2.7%: 95% CI = 0–7.9%) and Canada (4.7%: 95% CI = 0–10.9%). The French Research Group estimated that only 40% of twins with MS were registered with their database. Although it seems more likely that concordant monozygotic pairs would be overrepresented than underrepresented, this may not be the case. Even large population-based studies can be biased but, given that the French study is the only one among many to report a monozygotic twin concordance rate under 20%, the weight of evidence favours a monozygotic twin rate of at least 20%, which differs significantly from the rate for dizygotic twins.

Twin studies provide evidence that genetic susceptibility plays a role in the development of MS since monozygotic twins quite consistently have a higher concordance rate than dizygotic twins. However, these studies also provide one of the strongest arguments for an environmental cause because, even when the entire genotype of an MS twin is duplicated, the likelihood of that twin developing MS is still much less than 100%. The risk for dizygotic twins is only slightly higher than that for non-twin siblings. Rather than discounting an environmental factor, this may indicate that environmental sharing among dizygotic twins is not much more extensive than that among most non-twin siblings. In a single family with an inherited autosomal dominant neurological disease such as familial spastic paraparesis or some of the hereditary spinocerebellar degenerations, the age of onset of initial symptoms and the exact clinical profile and rate of progression may be quite variable over time in patients who presumably have the same genetic defect. Longitudinal twin studies using clinical features, MRI, and CSF immunochemistry would therefore be preferable in future research to establish concordance rates.

3.4.4 Adoptees and half-siblings

It has been argued that even the excess concordance in monozygotic twins compared with dizygotic twins and non-twin siblings could be attributed to increased environmental sharing. This issue has been addressed in genetic studies of various behavioural and psychiatric disorders, by looking at individuals adopted within 1 year of birth, comparing risks for patients' biological and adopted children raised in the same environment. If the etiological importance of genetics exceeds that of environment, the risk of MS in patients' biological children should be greater than that in their adopted children; the risk in adopted children should be similar to that in the general population. Conversely, if MS is determined by familial environment, the risk for adopted children would be the same as for biological children sharing the same environment. An intermediate risk for adopted children would suggest an interplay of genetics and family environment.

Like twin studies, adoptee studies are complicated by the need for a large population and unbiased case-ascertainment. Advertising for adoptees could presumably be subject to the same problems as advertising for subjects for many twin studies: in particular, MS patients whose adoptive parents have MS may be more likely to volunteer.

Only one population-based MS study of adoptees appears to have been published (Ebers, Sadovnick & Risch, 1995). Approximately 15 000 patients attending 14 regionally based MS clinics across Canada were surveyed to determine whether they were adopted and/or had non-biological first-degree relatives, including parents, siblings, and children. The time of adoption was defined as the date when adoptees began to live uninterruptedly with their adoptive families. MS patients adopted after the age of 1 year were excluded, as were individuals adopted by biological relatives. The survey identified 815 eligible patients (index cases) who had a total of 5055 biological and 1201 non-biological relatives. Lifetime age-adjusted recurrence risks and 95% CIs were calculated for biological relatives of these patients: for parents 2.0% (±0.35%); for siblings 3.6% (±0.50); and for children 2.7% (±1.09). No non-biological parent developed MS after adopting an index case, and no non-biological siblings or children of index cases developed the disease.

The findings of this study support a greater genetic than environmental contribution to the disease in that the risk for biological children of MS patients is greater than for non-biological children. However, the risk for non-biological children is essentially 0%—lower than the reported risk of 0.1% in the general population (Kurtzke, Beebe & Norman, 1985). This may indicate some underreporting of MS cases among adopted children; alternatively, the stipulation that a child must have been adopted by the age of 1 year may have been too strict, since migration studies suggest that some key environmental factor plays a role before age 15 and even more specifically at about age 12 (Kurtzke, Beebe & Norman, 1985). Ebers, Sadovnick & Risch (1995) do not report the number of adopted children identified after 1 year of age in the Canada-wide survey or their MS status. The risk of MS among adoptees of MS patients may need further clarification.

In a related study, Sadovnick et al. (1996) identified 939 people with MS who had half-siblings. The investigators found that the risk for half-siblings of developing MS, while less than that for full siblings, was greater than that for the general population. They also found no difference in risk of MS between half-siblings raised in the same household as individuals who later developed MS and those raised separately. Taking these findings together with the results of the adoptee study, the investigators suggested that the macroenvironment of the community, not the microenvironment of the family, is implicated in MS etiology.

3.4.5 Conjugal multiple sclerosis

Husbands and wives constitute another non-related group that has been studied for the effects of genetics versus environment. If exposure to an environmental risk factor during adult life were important, conjugal cases might be relatively common. Although there has been no systematic study large enough to permit definitive conclusions to be drawn about risk alteration for spouses of MS patients, available reports suggest that risk does not appear to be elevated. Millar & Allison (1954) found no conjugal MS pairs among 700 married patients, whereas McAlpine et al. (1955) found 3 among 1000 couples, Hyllested (1956) 1 among 2681 and Schapira, Poskanzer & Miller (1963) 1 among 608. Schapira, Poskanzer & Miller calculated the prevalence of MS among spouses of patients to be 4.9/10 000, which was similar to the rate of 5.0/10 000 in the general population of the English counties of Northumberland and Durham. The Canadian Collaborative Study on Genetic Susceptibility to Multiple Sclerosis recently confirmed that the risk for spouses of MS patients was no greater than for the general population (Sadovnick, 2000; personal communication). However, this observation does not necessarily support any contention that genetic factors determine familial aggregation, since a crucial environmental risk factor is thought to be operative before the age of 15 years—typically, therefore, before marriage.

With any mode of genetic transmission, the children of conjugal couples with MS should be at elevated risk. Cendrowski (1966) reported one case of MS in the only child of a conjugal couple. More recently Robertson & Compston (1995) examined recurrence risks in the children of 30 nationally recruited conjugal pairs of MS patients and found a risk of 6.8%—5 out of 73 children had clinically definite MS. The Canadian Collaborative Study also found that the risk for offspring when both parents have MS is 10 times that when only one parent has MS (Sadovnick, 2000; personal communication).

3.4.6 The role of genetics in the etiology of multiple sclerosis

It is now generally accepted that the etiology of MS involves some interplay of genetic and environmental factors. Evidence of racial or ethnic resistance, the increased risk among MS family members, and elevated monozygotic twin concordance rate all favour a genetic contribution to acquisition of the disease. However, the studies from which this evidence is derived also indicate that genetics cannot entirely explain the occurrence of MS. This is underlined by the fact that no population-based study of monozygotic twins has found a concordance rate in excess of 30%. Some environmental factor, such as a virus or toxin, must still play a role. This causal factor, and other enhancing or protective factors that influence the acquisition or impact of the causal factor or clinical manifestation of the disease, may be linked to genetics through the cultural environment. Just as environmental risk factors have yet to be identified, the role of genetics in MS remains to be clarified. That role is likely to be extensive and intricate, however, since the pattern of recurrence risks in families suggests that two or more susceptibility genes are involved. To date, only one of the candidate genes examined as susceptibility markers has withstood critical scrutiny, and that is the DR15 class 2 MHC allele association in northern Europeans (Compston et al., 1995; Chataway et al., 1998). There is no evidence that any genetic marker, acting alone or in combination, protects individuals from developing MS.

3.5 Other risk factors

Several other apparent MS risk factors have been explored for clues to etiology, including sex, age, trauma or emotional stress, and associated diseases. While their possible role in influencing environmental exposures has been considered, more attention has been paid to their potential influence on susceptibility.

3.5.1 Sex

Differences in the incidence of disease between the sexes are common and may or may not provide clues to etiology. The consistently higher occurrence of MS in women could reflect various factors, including genetic susceptibility, genetically-related immunological factors, hormonal influences, or environmental exposures.

A few researchers have suggested a relationship between sex and MS susceptibility based on genetics. Although X-linked recessive inheritance is incompatible with the sex ratio of affected cases, X-linked dominant inheritance would account for it, or a Y-linked resistance gene (or genes) could explain the sex ratio in MS. If susceptibility were related to sex, affected relatives would be more likely to have identical susceptibility genes, regardless of any specific inheritance pattern. The interaction between these genes and sex should result in a higher proportion of same-sex concordant relatives than expected. In support of this hypothesis, a literature review conducted by Weitkamp (1983) found that concordant MS siblings were more often of the same-sex than would be expected by chance. However, two population-based studies (Sadovnick et al., 1991; Warren & Warren, 1996) failed to confirm this observation.

Alternatively, a role for sex-linked factors in autoimmunity has been suggested because several autoimmune diseases, including Hashimoto disease, Crohn disease, myasthenia gravis, and systemic lupus erythmatosus, occur more frequently in women than in men. There is evidence of an association between alleles since the frequency of HLA-DR2b (DRB1*1501) is significantly higher in females than males (Van Lambalgen, Sanders & D'Amaro, 1986). Women may be more likely than men to inherit an allele that renders them susceptible to an environmental immunological stimulus associated with the development of MS.

A more popular theory is that the preponderance of women among MS patients reflects a hormonal factor that affects susceptibility. Androgens can suppress and estrogens enhance autoimmunity in diseases such as thyroiditis, myasthenia gravis, and polyarthritis. For example, estrogen influences a DNA sequence that stimulates nearby genes: the genes in turn transcribe interferon gamma, which helps to up-regulate the autoimmune system (Steinman, 1993). Although hormone levels remain relatively stable throughout the male lifespan, they change quite dramatically in females. The MS incidence curve is similar for men and women, except that incidence levels are higher in women. Researchers have therefore postulated that, although men may be equally exposed to an environmental factor, and that the chance of such exposure increases up to age 30 and then falls off, sex-linked hormones may increase women's susceptibility to the factor. In support of this theory, Duquette et al. (1987) have noted that the most dramatic preponderance of females with MS is evident around the age of puberty; incidence in women tends to converge with that in men after age 30, falling to its lowest point around menopause.

Van Lambalgen, Sanders & D'Amaro (1986) contend that clinical manifestations of the disease (that is, relapses) also parallel changes in the estrogen/luteinizing hormone balance during the menstrual cycle and after pregnancy. Epidemiological studies, frequently based on recall, have pursued this contention. At least one survey (McAlpine & Compston, 1952) has indicated that symptoms improve during menstruation and the first half of the menstrual cycle. Research has generally shown that the disease is relatively inactive during pregnancy compared with the postpartum period, although any minor increase in relapses during the puerperium may be due to the stress of labour or increased household responsibilities (Tillman, 1950; Sweeney, 1955; Millar et al., 1959; Schapira et al., 1966; Ghezzi & Caputo, 1981; Poser & Poser, 1983; Korn-Lubetzki et al., 1984; Nelson, Franklin & Jones, 1988; Sadovnick, 1994; Hours et al., 1995; Runmarker & Andersen, 1995). Two studies found no evidence that contraceptive use was associated with an increased number of exacerbations (Poser et al., 1979; Thorogood and Hannaford, 1998).

Finally, the preponderance of women among MS patients may indicate more frequent exposure to some environmental risk factor. Migration studies suggest that a crucial environmental factor may have its main impact around the time of puberty, but it is not immediately clear to what female children are more likely to be exposed than male children. Later in life, however, women may be more frequently exposed to causal factors or triggers associated either with domestic responsibilities (such as children with viral infections) or with certain occupations. For example, several of the female patients in the Key West cluster had worked as nurses (Helmick et al., 1989), and other studies have found an elevated MS risk among health care workers including doctors and nurses (Shepherd, 1991) or among nurses in particular (Lauer,

1995). Some researchers have speculated that exposure to chemicals associated with the hospital setting (Lauer, 1995) or microtraumatization of the cervical cord (Poser, 1987), which can occur during lifting and twisting activities performed by nurses, may play a role in the development of MS.

3.5.2 Age

Age–incidence curves for MS reported in both high- and low-risk countries world-wide are remarkably symmetrical and generally unimodal, which is atypical for a chronic disease. Cumulative exposure to an environmental risk factor usually results in an exponential rise in incidence, as illustrated by smoking and lung cancer. Instead, the MS age curve suggests that chance susceptibility or exposure to some environmental risk factor increases to a peak around age 30 and then decreases with age. A rapid decline in susceptibility occurs with age in acute viral infections, which confer lifelong immunity, but the age–incidence pattern of MS does not match that of any known viral disease (Brody, 1972). If MS is a long-delayed, rare consequence of a childhood infection that usually confers lifelong immunity, a decline in middle-age would be expected. In that case, however, the age–incidence curve or average age of onset should differ between countries where disease occurrence is low and those where it is high. If some causal infection is more common in high-risk areas, onset should peak at a younger age; or, if a causal infection is ubiquitous but later acquisition in high-risk areas is more likely to produce MS, onset should occur at a later age. In reality, neither pattern applies.

Although there is no clear evidence that MS occurrence varies with residence in urban or rural areas (Acheson, 1985), a few researchers have suggested that the age curve or average age of onset does vary with settings, which might imply a difference in exposure to some infection or other environmental risk factor. However, since some studies indicate earlier onset in urban areas (Alter, 1962; Detels et al., 1978) and others suggest earlier onset in rural areas (Poskanzer, Schapira & Miller, 1963a; Roberts, 1986), no clear pattern emerges.

It has also been suggested that age at onset varies with sex, in that MS incidence tends to reach a peak at a slightly earlier age in women than in men (Acheson, 1985; Van Lambalgen, Sanders & D'Amaro, 1986). Van Lambalgen, Sanders & D'Amaro (1986) have hypothesized that the etiology of MS is different for men and women, with hormonal factors playing a greater role in women and infections a greater role in men. However, there are several other possible explanations for earlier onset in women. It may be that women simply notice symptoms and seek medical attention sooner than men. Alternatively, the female:male ratio is higher for the RR form of MS, and onset of this form of the disease tends to be earlier than that of the CP form (Poser, Raun & Poser, 1982; Larsen et al., 1985)—a phenomenon that some researchers (Poser, Raun & Poser, 1982) have attributed to a decline in the immune system with age, which increases the impact of a triggering agent. When only RR patients were included in a risk factor study, Warren, Cockerill & Warren (1991) found that sex did not predict age of onset.

It is also unclear whether age of onset varies with race or ethnicity. Different age peaks for onset of MS have been observed in British and northern European immigrants to South Africa, with British immigrants developing the disease at an earlier age (Dean & Kurtzke, 1971). However, Acheson (1985) found no evidence of different age peaks for onset among immigrants to Israel, and Warren, Cockerill & Warren (1991) found no evidence that ethnicity was a factor for age of onset. If race or ethnicity does play a role in age of onset, it may be either through cultural environment or genetic susceptibility. Some researchers (Bulman et al., 1991) have suggested that age of onset of MS is partly under genetic control; they observed a correlation among sibling pairs concordant for MS, particularly when concordant monozygotic twin pairs were compared with non-twin sibling pairs. However, other researchers have not confirmed such an association (Warren & Warren, 1996).

3.5.3 Trauma and emotional stress

Clinical experience suggests that trauma or emotional stress may be associated with the onset of MS or with relapse (Acheson, 1985), and biologically plausible explanations have been advanced for both. Trauma might precipitate MS onset through overt damage to the CNS; conduction in demyelinated plaques is extremely sensitive to environmental change so that, as Poser (1987) has hypothesized, trauma may alter the safety factor in existing lesions to produce exacerbations. Several mechanisms have been suggested through which emotional stress may operate, including increased susceptibility to microbial infections (Dubos, 1965; Kaplan, 1975), impaired cell-mediated immunity (Rogers, Dubey & Reich, 1979), and altered hormone levels (Jacobs & Charles, 1980).

Trauma has been variously defined as including major physical trauma, head injury, fractures, surgery, and electric shock. There have been many uncontrolled studies of trauma and MS onset or relapse; most controlled studies have been retrospective and therefore subject to recall bias. The majority of controlled retrospective studies have found no relationship between trauma and MS onset (Alter & Speer, 1968; Von Wilhelm, 1970; Currier, Martin & Woosley, 1974; Bobowick et al., 1978; Bamford et al., 1981; Warren et al., 1982); only a few have found an association (Westlund & Kurland, 1953b; Poskanzer, 1965). At least two controlled retrospective studies (McAlpine & Compston, 1952; Warren, Warren & Cockerill, 1991) and two prospective studies (Sibley et al., 1991; Siva et al., 1993) have failed to find any association between trauma and relapse. In general, then, neither descriptive nor analytical studies suggest a relationship between trauma and the subsequent development or exacerbation of MS. Few forms of trauma are consistently followed by active MS disease and patients with MS do not consistently report a preceding history of physical stress or trauma of any kind.

The evidence that emotional stress may play a role in MS is more ambiguous. Again, most controlled studies have been retrospective and consequently subject not only to recall bias but also to ambiguity of cause and effect. The beginnings of both MS onset and relapses can be occult, making it difficult to establish whether stress precedes symptoms of the disease or undetected disease activity causes personality changes in patients that precipitate stressful events (for example, conflicts related to marriage, family, or employment). Several early retrospective studies found no obvious differences between patients and controls with regard to stress before onset (Braceland & Giffin, 1950) or revealed only inconclusive trends (Pratt, 1951; Baldwin, 1952; Alter et al., 1968). In a few later studies, however, significant differences were observed (Warren et al., 1982; Grant et al., 1989).

Retrospective studies that have examined whether stress precipitates relapse (by comparing patients in exacerbation with those in remission) have also produced conflicting results: two found no association (Rabins et al., 1986; Logsdail, Callanan & Ron, 1988), one a nonsignificant trend (Pratt, 1951), and two others a positive relationship (Dalos et al., 1983; Warren, Warren & Cockerill, 1991). Similarly, Franklin et al. (1988) observed in a prospective study that emotional stress was a risk factor for exacerbation of MS, while Sibley (1988) found no such association. Even when a positive association between emotional stress and MS onset or relapse has been found, the variance explained by stress is typically less than 10%.

3.5.4 Associated diseases

If a definite link could be established with some disease whose cause is better understood, it might provide clues to the etiology of MS. Because many researchers believe that MS is an autoimmune disease, both descriptive and analytical studies have focused on a possible association between MS and other autoimmune diseases. There is apparently no autoimmune disease that exhibits a global north–south gradient similar to that in MS, although this type of pattern has been reported for juvenile-onset insulin-dependent diabetes mellitus both within northern Europe (Rewers et al., 1988) and between countries throughout the world (Diabetes Epidemiology Research International Group, 1988).

Anecdotal evidence and small case series have suggested an association between MS and myasthenia gravis (Margolis & Graves, 1945; Aita, Snyder & Reichl, 1974; Achari, Trontelj & Campos, 1976; Shakir, Hussein & Trontelj, 1983), ankylosing spondylitis (Khan & Kushner, 1979), ulcerative colitis (Rang, Brooke & Hermon-Taylor, 1982; Minuk & Lewkonia, 1986), thyroid disease (Bixenman & Buchsbaum, 1988), and scleroderma (Trostle, Helfrich & Medsger, 1986). In two case–control studies with over 100 participants in each group, Warren & Warren (1981, 1982) observed that more MS patients were diabetic or reported a family history of diabetes than was the case among either neurological or normal controls. Wynn et al. (1990) found elevated relative risks for thyroid disease (Hashimoto thyroiditis and

Graves disease), diabetes mellitus, and rheumatoid arthritis among MS patients compared with the general population, but the differences were not statistically significant. Several other large studies that have compared patients (on personal or family history) with specific controls have likewise failed to confirm a statistically significant association between MS and diabetes or any other autoimmune disease (Hader, Elliot & Ebers, 1988; Rudez et al., 1995). However, Wertman, Zilber & Abramsky (1992) reported that the prevalence of insulin-dependent diabetes mellitus among 334 MS patients under the age of 30 in Israel was 8.98 per 1000, which was significantly higher than the rate for the same age group in the general population (0.095 per 1000).

3.6 Prognostic factors

Since some MS patients experience a benign disease course, there has been considerable interest in factors that might predict disability outcome. One of the principal methodological issues for prognostic studies is how to classify individual cases of the disease as benign or disabling. Researchers have defined various characteristics of patients with benign disease, including continued ability to work, full ambulatory abilities, and scores below a certain level on a scale such as the Expanded Disability Status Scale (Kurtzke, 1965). For their disease to be classified as benign according to any of these criteria, most researchers require that patients have had symptoms for at least 10 years, or that at least 10 years have elapsed since diagnosis; in some patients, however, the disease may remain benign for this period of time and subsequently become progressively disabling (Matthews, 1985). Estimates of the percentage of patients who eventually become disabled vary somewhat, largely because of differences in the researchers' disability classification criteria and on whether they combine cases with an RR onset with primary CP cases in their analysis.

A few studies, either retrospective or prospective, have examined long-term prognosis in a relatively large group of patients. McAlpine (1961) reported that disease remained benign in approximately 33% of patients with RR MS 10 years after onset, in 25% 15 years after onset, and in 20% 20 years after onset. The definition of benign disease required that a patient was able to walk half a mile (about 800 metres) without assistance and was still working away from or within the home. Percy et al. (1971) found that about 65% of RR patients who survived for more than 25 years remained ambulant. Benedikz (1994) reported that disease remained benign in 85% of MS patients (on the basis of a low-end score on the Expanded Disability Status Scale) after 5 years, compared with 38% after 20 years, when RR and CP cases were combined. When these groups were separated, the figures for RR patients were 98% after 5 years and 63% after 30 years, compared with only 60% for CP patients after 5 years and 10% after 25 years. Myhr et al. (1994) reported that 58% of RR and 68% of CP patients were collecting a disability pension after 19 years and that, of the CP patients, 86% needed assistance to walk and 75% were using a wheelchair. Although percentages of patients in these series whose disease remains benign vary, they uniformly decline with disease duration. Patient and disease characteristics that predict outcome have been identified, but possible environmental or genetic factors remain relatively unexplored.

3.6.1 Patient and disease characteristics

Early analytical studies that examined which patient and disease characteristics predict disability outcome among MS patients have been reviewed by a number of authors (Kraft et al., 1981; Hallpike, 1983; Acheson, 1985), and their results have been generally confirmed by some more recent work (Runmarker & Andersen, 1993; Italian Multicentre Collaborative Group, 1994; Kruja, 1994; Myhr et al., 1994; Hernandez et al., 1995; Kantarci et al., 1998; Amato et al., 1999; Hawkins & McDonnell, 1999; Levic et al., 1999). Despite some minor variability in results, there is good general agreement on characteristics associated with a benign course:

— early onset
— primary RR course
— monosymptomatic onset
— visual or sensory first symptoms
— absence of motor or cerebellar signs
— rapid remission after first symptom
— long interval between first and second relapse
— low relapse frequency in early years
— little or no residual deficit and the absence of pyramidal or cerebellar involvement after 5 years.

Studies that have observed a difference by sex usually indicate that males experience a more severe course (Muller, 1949; Panelius, 1969; Detels et al., 1982; Warren et al., 1985b; Duquette et al., 1987; Runmarker & Andersen, 1993; Myhr et al., 1994; Kantarci et al., 1998; Hawkins & McDonnell, 1999; Levic et al., 1999).

3.6.2 Environmental and genetic factors

Although fewer in number, prognostic studies have concentrated on the same environmental and genetic factors as risk studies. The effect of latitude has been studied most often, with variable results. In a study comparing high-risk Winnipeg, Canada, with low-risk New Orleans, USA, no difference was found in the rate of progression to disability (Stazio, Paddison & Kurland, 1967). Patients in medium-risk Charleston, USA, had only a slight tendency towards greater disability than those in high-risk Halifax, Canada (Alter et al., 1960). By contrast, substantial differences have been noted in a number of studies carried out in a variety of settings, including Australia (Hammond et al., 1988b), Europe (Prange et al., 1986), and the USA (Detels et al., 1982). In the Australian study greater disability (among males only) was observed in the warmer region of Queensland than in more southern areas of

Australia. This confirmed the results of a prospective study in the USA, in which progression to disease was compared in MS patients from the state of Washington with patients from Los Angeles, California (Detels et al., 1982). Although patients in both areas had a similar mean age of onset, and a similar distribution by diagnostic category at recruitment, patients in low-risk Los Angeles experienced a more disabling course.

A worse prognosis in low-risk areas may indicate that some factor that decreases the risk of acquiring the disease paradoxically increases the chance of disability. Several studies have observed a clinical relationship between exposure to heat and temporary exacerbation of symptoms (Acheson, 1985). Patients in warmer climates may experience more frequent and prolonged exacerbations than patients in colder climates, although no empirical evidence supports this hypothesis.

Remarkably, there appear to be almost no retrospective or prospective studies of other possible environmental or genetic predictors. Warren et al. (1985b) compared patients who were still classified as benign 10 years after onset with disabled patients on a variety of lifestyle factors/experiences, including diet, vitamin, alcohol and tobacco use, physical activity, emotional stress, pregnancy, urban/rural residence, socioeconomic status, and other illnesses. None of these variables was associated with disability. Moreover, patients with benign disease were no more likely than others to report a family history of MS but were more likely to report diabetes in their families. A greater percentage of these patients reported northern European, rather than British, ancestry, although this difference was not statistically significant.

Other research has confirmed that neither pregnancy (Ghezzi & Caputo, 1981; Runmarker & Andersen, 1995) nor a family history of MS (Matthews, 1985; Weinshenker et al., 1990) is associated with greater disability, but the role of other possible predictors has yet to be clarified. Recently McDonnell et al. (1999) examined whether DR alleles influenced prognosis; they found no single DR allele to be associated with either a good or a poor prognosis. On the other hand, Fukazawa et al. (1999) observed that clinical disability was significantly more severe in AA homozygous Japanese MS patients. Brassat et al. (1999) found similar disease progression in 87 concordant MS sibling pairs, concluding that disability might be influenced by familial factors (environmental or genetic).

4.
Temporal trends

Examination of frequency trends worldwide may provide clues to the cause of MS. The patterns of geographical distribution, together with data from migrant studies, suggest that environmental factors are etiologically important and that there is a latency between exposure and onset of disease. At any point in time, geographical variation in the prevalence or incidence of MS may be due to variation in environmental exposure to a causal factor. Similarly, changes in prevalence or incidence rates over time can be examined to determine whether they resemble temporal patterns of exposure to a possible causal factor. For example, Swank (1961) has argued that increasing MS prevalence during the 20th century may be related to increased consumption of animal fats deficient in unsaturated fatty acids. In the case of incidence, some researchers who postulated a role for measles in the etiology of MS predicted a decline in the occurrence in the USA during the 1990s as a result of the widespread immunization of children against measles that began around 1965 (Nathanson, 1980). Of possibly greater interest are fluctuations in incidence, such as the apparent correlation (taking into account lag time) between cyclical outbreaks of canine distemper and peaks in MS incidence observed in the province of Newfoundland, Canada (Pryse-Phillips, 1986). Fluctuating incidence rates favour the idea of an environmental causal factor because it is difficult to see how genetically determined disease could manifest itself cyclically.

The prevalence of MS has clearly increased during the 1900s. Whether this trend reflects increasing incidence, longer survival, changes in diagnostic criteria and case-ascertainment, or population shifts in various geographical regions, remains open to debate.

4.1 Changes in the prevalence of multiple sclerosis

Early case reports indicate that MS existed in France, Germany, the United Kingdom, and the USA at least as early as the 19th century. The first generally accepted clinical description (Firth, 1948) is the case of Auguste d'Este, a grandson of King George III and nephew of Queen Victoria, who chronicled his own condition from its onset in 1822. Jean Martin Charcot, a professor at the Faculty of Medicine of Paris, is usually acknowledged as the first physician to systematically describe the clinical features and pathological alterations associated with MS in medical lectures published in 1877 (Wechsler, 1953; Guillain, 1959). However, Charcot attributed the earliest clinical and pathological descriptions of the disease to a former professor, Jean Cruveilhier, in 1835 (Bourneville, 1892). Frerichs published a report in 1849 that detailed the histories of several German patients whose clinical descriptions conform to current concepts, including the RR course that may gradually progress to paralysis. The first documented cases of MS in England—eight young adult patients with a typical clinical course—were reported by Moxon (1875). Seguin, Shaw & Van Derveer (1878) are credited with the initial American description of MS in two patients whose symptoms and disease course were consistent with the recognized pattern.

Some researchers have speculated that MS existed far earlier in Europe. Medaer (1979) has described a Dutch woman, Lidvina van Schiedam, living in the 13th century, whose disease began when she was 16 and was characterized by paralysis of both legs and her right arm, facial palsy, bilateral loss of vision, sensory changes, and dysphagia over the next 37 years. Poser (1995) has suggested that MS may also have occurred in Iceland as early as the 1200s, citing the case of a woman named Halla who became ill and then recovered, supposedly through the intercession of St Thorlakr, from symptoms that may have represented a first attack of MS.

Regardless of when it first occurred, MS was certainly well known in the international medical literature by the end of the 19th century. However, its prevalence was not systematically studied until the 1900s, so that its frequency in Europe, the USA, and other areas of the world before the 20th century remains unknown. Many recent studies, however, provide a detailed picture of the current prevalence of MS worldwide, and a few of these also specifically address the issue of whether prevalence is increasing.

To examine changes in prevalence over time, some surveys have been conducted in different regions of a particular country at different points in time. Many of these indicate prevalence has indeed risen over the years. Williams, Jones & McKeran (1991), for example, compared prevalence rates collected throughout England in the 1950s with those collected in the 1980s, noting that figures for the 1980s were substantially higher. Surveys conducted in various Italian cities between the late 1960s and mid-1970s indicated prevalence rates ranging from 10 to 20 per 100 000 population. Later surveys, in the late 1970s and 1980s, produced rates in the order of 31 to 90 per 100 000, leading some researchers to change the classification of Italy from medium to high risk (Kurtzke, 1991). Prevalence studies conducted throughout several Canadian provinces from the mid-20th century onwards also tended to find increasing prevalence rates: before the 1980s rates averaged 42/ 100 000 and have since risen to125/100 000. However, only limited conclusions can be drawn from such comparisons, since higher rates in more recently studied regions may reflect geographical variations rather than increases in prevalence. The relatively low rate of 55/100 000 observed in Newfoundland (Pryse-Phillips, 1986)—

one of the most recently surveyed provinces—illustrates this possibility. Like all the Canadian provinces, Newfoundland has distinct characteristics that may be related to MS etiology.

Fewer prevalence studies have been conducted over time in particular regions. Table 7 illustrates the findings of 25 such studies, including those conducted in Australia (Perth; Newcastle; Hobart); Bulgaria (Sofia); Canada (Winnipeg; Saskatoon); Denmark and the Faeroe Islands; Finland (Turku); Iceland; Italy (Ferrara; L'Aquila) and Sardinia (Barbagia; Nuoro); Northern Ireland; Norway (More and Romsdal; Hordaland; Troms and Finnmark); Poland (west); Scotland (Orkney Islands; Shetland Islands; Grampian region); Switzerland; the USA (Rochester; New Orleans). With the notable exceptions of Winnipeg, the Faeroe Islands, the Orkney Islands, and western Poland, these areas have all shown increases in MS prevalence over time, which may be due to a variety of factors other than increasing incidence of the disease.

Since prevalence is a function of both incidence and disease duration, longer survival is one possible explanation of rising prevalence rates. Kurtzke (1991) has suggested that MS mortality rates are decreasing worldwide and that more patients may be dying from other illnesses whose occurrence tends to increase with age. Because these are unrelated to MS, it may be that MS is not listed as an underlying cause of death. However, an examination of survival studies does not indicate any obvious trend towards longer MS duration over the past two decades, even though this would have been expected with better medical care (Matthews, 1985; Wynn et al., 1990; Midgard, Riise & Nyland, 1991). Recent studies from countries such as Canada (Warren et al., 1999[1]) and Denmark (Koch-Henriksen, 1995) indicate that mortality has not actually decreased but that it may fluctuate over time. Increases in both countries have been observed since the early 1990s.

Diagnostic criteria may also influence prevalence rates. Less stringent criteria could account for increases in prevalence, especially when "possible" cases are included and no distinction is made between overall rates and rates for probable/definite cases only. For example, the rates reported in Cambridge (Mumford et al., 1992), South Glamorgan (Swingler & Compston, 1988), and Southampton (Roberts et al., 1991) using the criteria of Allison & Millar (1954) were respectively 130, 117, and 99 per 100 000 when "possibles" were included, but uniformly lower at 107, 84, and 92 per 100 000 when they were excluded. Most recent studies, however, have used the criteria of either Schumacher et al. (1965) or Poser et al. (1983), both of which eliminate "possible" cases. Where they are available, the introduction of sophisticated laboratory tests such as MRI, which lead to earlier diagnosis and more likely diagnosis of benign disease, may contribute to increases in prevalence.

---

[1] *Mortality rates for multiple sclerosis in Canada.* Paper presented at the Regional North American Annual Meeting of the World Federation of Neurology—Research Group on Neuroepidemiology, Toronto.

Table 7. Trends in prevalence of multiple sclerosis

Country and/or region	Year or period	Prevalence per 100 000 pop.	References
United States			
Rochester, MN	1915	46	Percy et al. (1971)
	1978	108	Kranz et al. (1983)
	1985	173	Wynn et al. (1990)
New Orleans, LA	1950	10	Stazio, Paddison & Kurland (1967)
	1960	9	Stazio, Paddison & Kurland (1967)
Switzerland	1918–1922	23	Ackerman (1931)
	1956	51	Georgi et al. (1961)
	1986	52	Kesselring & Beer (1994)
Canada			
Winnipeg, Manitoba	1939–1948	40	Westlund & Kurland (1953b)
	1960	35	Stazio et al. (1964)
Saskatoon, Saskatchewan	1977	177	Hader (1982)
	1998	248	Hader (1999)
Faeroe Islands	1940	0	Kurtzke & Hyllested (1986)
	1950	47	Kurtzke & Hyllested (1986)
	1960	67	Kurtzke & Hyllested (1986)
	1970	54	Kurtzke & Hyllested (1986)
	1980	39	Kurtzke & Hyllested (1986)
Denmark (mainland)	1948	88	McAlpine (1985)
	1964	101	McAlpine (1985)
	1990	112	Koch-Henriksen (1999)
Northern Ireland	1951	41	McDonnell & Hawkins (1998)
	1961	57	McDonnell & Hawkins (1998)
	1986	104	McDonnell & Hawkins (1998)
	1998	191	McDonnell & Hawkins (1998)
Scotland			
Orkney Islands	1954	82	Poskanzer et al. (1980a)
	1962	167	Poskanzer et al. (1980a)
Shetland Islands	1970	222	Poskanzer et al. (1980a)
	1974	258	Poskanzer et al. (1980a)
	1983	193	Cook et al. (1985)
Grampian region	1954	118	Poskanzer et al. (1980a)
	1962	120	Poskanzer et al. (1980a)
	1970	131	Poskanzer et al. (1980a)
	1974	152	Poskanzer et al. (1980a)
	1983	170	Cook et al. (1988)
	1970	106	Phadke & Downie (1987)
	1980	145	Phadke & Downie (1987)
Iceland	1955	33	Poser, Benedikz & Hibberd (1992)
	1965	34	Poser, Benedikz & Hibberd (1992)
	1975	52	Poser, Benedikz & Hibberd (1992)
	1985	70	Poser, Benedikz & Hibberd (1992)
Australia			
Perth, WA	1961	19	McCall et al. (1968)
	1981	30	Hammond et al. (1988a)
Newcastle, NSW	1961	19	McCall et al. (1968)
	1981	37	Hammond et al. (1988a)
Hobart, Tas.	1961	33	McCall et al. (1968)
	1981	76	Hammond et al. (1988a)

Table 7. Continued

Country and/or region	Year or period	Prevalence per 100 000 pop.	References
Norway			
More and Romsdal	1961	24	Midgard, Riise & Nyland (1991)
	1985	75	Midgard, Riise & Nyland (1991)
Hordaland	1963	20	Larsen et al. (1984a)
	1983	60	Larsen et al. (1984a)
Troms and Finnmark	1973	21	Grønning & Mellgren (1985)
	1983	32	Grønning & Mellgren (1985)
Finland			
Turku	1964	30	Kinnunen (1984)
	1979	93	Kinnunen (1984)
Poland (western)	1965	51	Cendrowski et al. (1969)
	1981	43	Wender et al. (1985)
Italy			
Ferrara	1965	21	Granieri et al. (1985)
	1978	37	Granieri et al. (1985)
	1981	46	Granieri et al. (1985)
	1986	51	Granieri & Tola (1994)
	1993	68	Granieri & Tola (1994)
L'Aquila	1984	33	D'Aurizio et al. (1988)
	1996	53	Totaro et al. (2000)
Barbagia, Sardinia	1975	41	Granieri et al. (1983)
	1981	65	Granieri et al. (1983)
Nuoro, Sardinia	1985	103	Casetta et al. (1998)
	1993	144	Casetta et al. (1998)
Bulgaria			
Sofia	1992	30	Georgiev et al. (1994)
	1995	39	Milanov (1997)

Case-ascertainment methods may also lead to increased prevalence rates. Recognition of the limitations of individual data sources, such as death certificates, has encouraged researchers to broaden their efforts to identify cases. Improvements both in the neurological services in some countries and in the diagnostic abilities of clinicians—who may be identifying cases directly, or indirectly through record review—have probably increased patient identification. Wider public awareness of the disease and improved medical coverage encourage people to seek diagnosis and treatment and may also have brought more patients into the records of facilities through which cases are sought. When Hader (1982) first reported a prevalence rate exceeding 100/100 000 in Saskatoon, Canada, researchers initially speculated that specific MS risk factors might be more common in Saskatoon. Subsequently, Sadovnick & Ebers (1993) suggested that the Saskatoon rate was higher than had been found in previous surveys in other Canadian provinces because Hader was the only researcher in recent years whose study was specifically designed to determine prevalence; study results would therefore have been affected by changes bearing on case-ascertainment, including the implementation of universal medical care coverage. Their claim is supported by the observation that most Canadian prevalence studies conducted since then have also produced rates close to or exceeding 100/100 000. The highest rates in Canada come from Alberta and may be inflated because they were based on Alberta Health Care Insurance Plan records, which probably include charges for treatment of suspected, possible, or even misdiagnosed cases (Svenson, Woodhead & Platt, 1994). Recently Hader (1999) has presented evidence of a substantial rise in Saskatoon's prevalence rate, so that it is now similar to reported Alberta rates. This rise seems unlikely to be due solely to case-ascertainment since many of the major changes would have occurred by the 1980s.

In some instances, changes in case-ascertainment methods can lead to a *decrease* in prevalence rates. For example, the decline in Winnipeg from 40/100 000 for the years 1939–1948 to 35/100 000 in 1961 may have been largely a function of the means by which cases were identified for inclusion. The initial study was based on patient records and death certificates. In the follow-up survey (Stazio et al., 1964), 144 patients from the first study were diagnostically re-evaluated. Re-evaluation confirmed MS in only 78% of the 109 patients classified as "probable" in the first study. Of the remaining 24 patients, 6.4% were reclassified as "possible" MS and the other 15.6% as either unlikely or as definitely not having MS. Generally, however, re-evaluations of this nature are probably more likely to add cases who existed at the time of previous surveys but were not counted because patients' symptoms were insufficient for diagnosis. For example, prevalence rates in Iceland based on diagnosed cases were 33, 34, 52, and 70 per 100 000 for the years 1955, 1965, 1975, and 1985 respectively; rates based on date of onset for diagnosed cases were 59, 58, 67, and 79 per 100 000, indicating a less steep rise (Poser CM, 1994). To overcome this problem, Poser has suggested adopting the concept of the Onset-Adjusted Prevalence Rate, obtained by retrospectively counting individuals in whom disease onset occurred before the date for which prevalence is calculated but who are diagnosed subsequently. Most prevalence studies reported to date have not incorporated such a correction, but the possible implications should be kept in mind when increases in prevalence are assessed.

Finally, population shifts can account for apparent changes in prevalence. The age structure of a population can have a variety of effects: for example, a significant change in the number of people in high-risk age groups may account for observed changes in prevalence. In western Poland, an increase in the percentage of the population under age 20 (a low-risk group) may have resulted in the observed decrease in MS prevalence (Wender et al., 1985). Similarly, changes in the racial or ethnic composition of a population that influence genetic susceptibility may lead to rate increases or decreases.

Nonetheless, changes in incidence rather than any of the above factors may still contribute to real changes in prevalence. The Faeroe Islands outbreak has been classified as a point-source epidemic, possibly resulting from the introduction and withdrawal of some transmissible etiological agent, reflected in prevalence increases before 1960 and subsequent decreases.

4.2 Is the incidence of multiple sclerosis increasing?

Although most studies indicate an increase in the prevalence of MS, it is not clear that increasing incidence has contributed to this trend. Surveys conducted in different regions of a single country at different points in time indicate that incidence, like prevalence, is increasing, but higher rates in regions studied more recently may reflect geographical variation. Table 8 summarizes the results of several repeat surveys in the same geographical region. Conflicting patterns emerge, with some areas apparently stable and a few showing declines; in other areas, incidence rates have tended to increase over time. Regardless of the overall trend, many areas exhibit cyclical fluctuations. When rates are compared statistically, however, differences often fail to reach statistical significance, which could be interpreted to mean that MS rates are in fact generally stable.

Diagnostic criteria, case-ascertainment methods, and population shifts can operate to create changes in incidence over time in the same region, just as with prevalence. The recent development of MRI testing has significantly improved diagnostic accuracy in cases of benign MS; it may be this improvement, rather than a true increase in the disease itself, that explains apparent increases in incidence. In addition, many incidence rates are based on retrospectively collected onset data: that is, recorded dates of disease onset are used to calculate incidence. Because the onset of first symptoms can be difficult to identify, the recorded years of onset may be inaccurate and result in misleading patterns.

Misclassification can be particularly problematic for a disease with such low incidence—shift of even one case from numerator to denominator can have a considerable impact on incidence rates. Some researchers have argued, however, that there is no reason to believe that misclassification is so unevenly distributed as to create apparent fluctuations. Date of diagnosis is preferred by some investigators, but variable diagnostic criteria and changing lag periods from disease onset to diagnosis may result in apparent, but not real, differences. For example, the decreasing lag time between onset and diagnosis (Benedikz, Magnusson & Guthmundsson, 1994) might artificially create the impression that the incidence of MS is increasing in younger age groups within a population. Like prevalence rates, incidence rates based on diagnosis can be adjusted for age of onset (Hibberd, 1994). If the study aims to compare rates before and after time-specific exposures (such as the occupation of the Faeroe Islands by foreign military personnel), the fixed population present at the start of the exposure is examined to determine the number of patients with signs and symptoms of the disease within a reasonable incubation period (5–10 years). The cumulative incidence after exposure is compared with the cumulative incidence in a similar fixed

Table 8. Trends in incidence of multiple sclerosis[a]

Country and/or region	Year or period	Incidence per 100 000 pop.	References
Northern Ireland	1901–1905	1.0	Millar (1972)
	1906–1910	1.2	Millar (1972)
	1911–1915	1.1	Millar (1972)
	1916–1920	1.1	Millar (1972)
	1921–1925	1.1	Millar (1972)
	1985–1992	6.5	McDonnell & Hawkins (1998)
United States			
Rochester, MN	1905–1914	2.8	Wynn et al. (1990)
	1915–1924	2.9	Wynn et al. (1990)
	1925–1934	5.2	Wynn et al. (1990)
	1935–1944	2.3	Wynn et al. (1990)
	1945–1954	6.5	Wynn et al. (1990)
	1955–1964	4.9	Wynn et al. (1990)
	1965–1974	7.4	Wynn et al. (1990)
	1975–1984	6.3	Wynn et al. (1990)
Olmstead County, MN	1905–1914	1.2	Wynn et al. (1990)
	1915–1924	1.4	Wynn et al. (1990)
	1925–1934	3.5	Wynn et al. (1990)
	1935–1944	2.4	Wynn et al. (1990)
	1945–1954	5.3	Wynn et al. (1990)
	1955–1964	4.4	Wynn et al. (1990)
	1965–1974	7.9	Wynn et al. (1990)
	1975–1984	6.2	Wynn et al. (1990)
New Orleans, LA	1940–1949	.45	Stazio, Paddison & Kurland (1967)
	1950–1959	.39	Stazio, Paddison & Kurland (1967)
Sardinia			
Macomer	1912–1952	0	Rosati et al. (1986)
	1952–1981	13 cases	Rosati et al. (1986)
Barbagia	1961–1970	2.7	Granieri et al. (1983)
	1971–1980	3.1	Granieri et al. (1983)
Sassari	1965–1975	2.1	Rosati et al. (1988)
	1976–1985	4.6	Rosati et al. (1988)
Alghero	1971	1.6	Rosati et al. (1987)
	1980	5.9	Rosati et al. (1987)
Denmark	1939–1945	3.4	Hyllested (1956)
	1950–1959	5.1	Koch-Henriksen, Bronnum-Hansen & Hyllested (1992)
	1960–1969	3.9	Koch-Henriksen, Bronnum-Hansen & Hyllested (1992)
	1970–1979	4.3	Koch-Henriksen, Bronnum-Hansen & Hyllested (1992)
	1980–1989	4.9	Koch-Henriksen et al. (1999)
Canada			
Winnipeg, Manitoba	1940–1949	1.6	Stazio et al. (1964)
	1950–1959	1.5	Stazio et al. (1964)
Saskatoon, Saskatchewan	1950–1959	5.7	Hader (1982)
	1960–1969	4.1	Hader (1982)
	1970–1979	8.3	Hader (1999)
	1980–1989	9.2	Hader (1999)
Barrhead County, Alberta	1950–1959	4.3	Warren & Warren (1992)
	1960–1969	4.9	Warren & Warren (1992)
	1970–1979	3.8	Warren & Warren (1992)
	1980–1989	4.2	Warren & Warren (1992)
Westlock County, Alberta	1950–1959	1.9	Warren & Warren (1993)
	1960–1969	2.9	Warren & Warren (1993)
	1970–1979	3.8	Warren & Warren (1993)
	1980–1989	7.3	Warren & Warren (1993)

Table 8. Continued

Country and/or region	Year or period	Incidence per 100 000 pop.	References
Newfoundland	1960–1964	1.1	Pryse-Phillips (1986)
	1965–1969	1.9	Pryse-Phillips (1986)
	1970–1974	2.4	Pryse-Phillips (1986)
	1975–1979	2.8	Pryse-Phillips (1986)
	1980–1982	3.0	Pryse-Phillips (1986)
Scotland			
Orkney Islands	1940–1944	12.0	Cook et al. (1985)
	1945–1949	9.4	Cook et al. (1985)
	1950–1954	11.3	Cook et al. (1985)
	1955–1959	8.5	Cook et al. (1985)
	1960–1964	8.5	Cook et al. (1985)
	1965–1982	3.7	Cook et al. (1985)
Shetland Islands	1940–1944	9.1	Cook et al. (1988)
	1945–1949	11.4	Cook et al. (1988)
	1950–1954	4.1	Cook et al. (1988)
	1955–1959	9.0	Cook et al. (1988)
	1960–1964	3.4	Cook et al. (1988)
	1965–1969	8.1	Cook et al. (1988)
	1970–1986	5.3	Cook et al. (1988)
Grampian region	1960	4.6	Phadke & Downie (1987)
	1980	7.2	Phadke & Downie (1987)
Australia			
Perth, WA	1950–1959	1.2	Hammond et al. (1988a)
	1971–1981	1.3	Hammond et al. (1988a)
Hobart, Tas.	1950–1959	1.2	Hammond et al. (1988a)
	1971–1981	2.1	Hammond et al. (1988a)
Newcastle, NSW	1950–1959	2.2	Hammond et al. (1988a)
	1971–1981	3.5	Hammond et al. (1988a)
Norway			
More and Romsdal	1950–1954	1.7	Midgard, Riise & Nyland (1991)
	1955–1959	2.1	Midgard, Riise & Nyland (1991)
	1960–1964	1.7	Midgard, Riise & Nyland (1991)
	1965–1969	2.4	Midgard, Riise & Nyland (1991)
	1970–1974	1.8	Midgard, Riise & Nyland (1991)
	1975–1979	3.4	Midgard, Riise & Nyland (1991)
	1980–1984	2.0	Midgard, Riise & Nyland (1991)
Hordaland	1953–1957	1.8	Grønning et al. (1991)
	1958–1962	2.2	Grønning et al. (1991)
	1963–1967	2.8	Grønning et al. (1991)
	1968–1972	3.9	Grønning et al. (1991)
	1973–1977	4.1	Grønning et al. (1991)
	1978–1982	4.7	Grønning et al. (1991)
	1983–1987	3.2	Grønning et al. (1991)
Troms and Finnmark	1953–1978	1.8	Grønning & Mellgren (1985)
	1974–1982	1.9	Grønning & Mellgren (1985)
Sweden			
Gothenburg	1950–1954	4.2	Svenningson et al. (1990)
	1955–1959	4.2	Svenningson et al. (1990)
	1960–1964	4.3	Svenningson et al. (1990)
	1974–1978	3.0	Svenningson et al. (1990)
	1979–1983	2.7	Svenningson et al. (1990)
	1983–1988	2.0	Svenningson et al. (1990)
Germany			
Rostock	1963–1968	4.5	Kurtzke (1991)
	1969–1973	1.8	Kurtzke (1991)
	1974–1978	3.7	Kurtzke (1991)
	1979–1983	1.8	Kurtzke (1991)

did correct for delay in ascertainment. As a basis for the correction, the year of diagnosis was noted for all patients, allowing the latency period to be estimated for both sexes in three groups of age of onset (<25, 25–39, ±40). The incidence rates were corrected by dividing the incidence estimates for a specific year by the sex- and age-specific probabilities of cases being ascertained by 1986 (the correcting factor). Koch-Henriksen, Bronnum-Hansen & Hyllested (1992) report that the effect of correcting for delay of ascertainment was minimal in the first half of the study period, but notable from 1970 onward. Even after correction, the crude incidence rate for Denmark declined significantly from the 1950s to the 1960s. There appeared to be a slight increase in the 1970s compared with the 1960s, but the researchers suggested that the correction for delayed ascertainment in the 1970s may have been an overcompensation considering contemporary improvements in diagnosis and case-ascertainment. Nevertheless, the most recent adjusted assessment (Esberg, Keiding & Koch-Henriksen, 1999) confirms an increase.

Most geographical regions that exhibit increasing or decreasing trends in incidence, or even stable rates, also exhibit some cyclical ups and downs. It has been suggested that Newfoundland has shown a more definite cyclic pattern than other regions (Pryse-Phillips, 1986), although this assertion seems to be based on peaks observed in 1965, 1970, 1976, and 1981, rather than over the five-year intervals shown in Table 8. The most clear-cut, statistically significant fluctuating pattern was identified for Rostock in the former German Democratic Republic: incidence fell by 2.7 per 100 000 for the period 1969–1973 compared with 1963–1968, rose by 1.9 for the period 1974–1978, and fell again by 1.9 for the period 1979–1983 (Meyer-Rienecker & Buddenhagen, 1988). Since the end of observations in 1984, Kurtzke (1991) has commented that the final decline may be the result of delayed case-ascertainment but accepts that the previous decline is probably real.

Several authors have concluded that the variable patterns in incidence rates, particularly cyclic fluctuations independent of the general trend, implicate an environmental factor in the etiology of MS. This argument is further supported by the fact that fluctuations have been reported by many countries even during the years before any major advances in diagnosis and case-ascertainment, that is, pre-1970. The most popular theory is that the cyclic pattern of incidence is tied to variations in the presence of a transmissible agent, since environmental factors such as diet, housing, and sanitation tend to improve over time while factors like climate remain relatively stable.

4.3 Changes in the clinical picture of multiple sclerosis

Some studies that have shown an increase in MS incidence indicate that this has occurred predominantly among females. In Newfoundland, for example, incidence rates for males in the province as a whole remained stable whereas rates for females showed an impressive and continuing increase (Pryse-Phillips, 1986). Kinnunen

78

(1984) observed the same pattern in Finland for both Uusimaa and Vaasa provinces. In Uusimaa the incidence rates for males were 1.8, 1.8, and 1.2 per 100 000 and for females 2.2, 3.5, and 2.5 over the periods 1964–1968, 1969–1973, and 1974–1978 respectively, with the female : male ratio changing from 1.2 : 1 to 2 : 1 over time. This pattern was even more noticeable in Vaasa where the rates for males were 3.2, 3.1 and 1.9 per 100 000 but 3.1, 4.1 and 4.2 for females, with the female : male ratio changing from 1 : 1 to 2.2 : 1. Similar differences in the incidence patterns for males and females have been reported in Hordaland (Grønning et al., 1991) and the northern part of Norway (Grønning & Mellgren, 1985).

In Hordaland, there also appears to have been a greater increase in the incidence of MS that is initially RR rather than CP (Grønning et al., 1991), although the difference did not quite reach statistical significance. Since it has been suggested that women experience a more benign form of the disease than men (Van Lambalgen, Sanders & D'Amaro, 1986), an apparent increase in the RR form may be related to an increased incidence of MS in women. However, improved diagnostic criteria and case-ascertainment may mean that cases of remitting disease have simply been recognized earlier in recent years, creating the impression of a disparity.

5.
Conclusions and challenges for future research

After more than a century of epidemiological research, many questions still remain about the distribution of MS, risk of the disease, and prognostic factors. It may be that the relevant etiological variables have not yet been studied. On the other hand, the failure to identify important exposures may be explained by methodological issues in areas that include: diagnostic criteria, low disease frequency, apparently different influences on acquisition and clinical manifestation, difficulty in identifying appropriate "windows" of exposure, retrospective versus prospective studies, and the possibility that the disease exists in more than one form. Other potential areas of research, such as prenatal risk factors, have received little attention.

5.1 Diagnostic criteria

The adoption of consistent diagnostic criteria would increase the accuracy of future comparisons of disease frequency between and within regions over time. On the basis of apparent acceptance, the criteria developed by Poser et al. (1983) seem to be the most promising. In a recent survey on the use of various classification systems in European studies of MS prevalence, Rosati (1994) found that only one study used the criteria of McDonald & Halliday (1977), two used those of Rose et al. (1976), seven Allison & Millar (1954), 11 Schumacher et al. (1965), three McAlpine (1985), four Bauer (1980), and 25 Poser et al. (1983). An additional benefit of using the criteria of Poser et al. would be the elimination of "possible" cases. This would help to avoid misclassification of patients, which could inflate frequency values or mask the effect of risk factors in analytical studies. Even if these criteria were to be generally adopted, however, some reliability and validity testing of the system would be useful. In studies that count patients recorded in treatment facility files, the use of a uniform, coded diagnostic index—such as that provided by ICD-10—would promote comparability of incidence and prevalence rates.

5.2 Low frequency

Large patient pools are needed to identify sufficient cases of MS to allow certain research questions to be addressed. For a disease as relatively uncommon as MS, the multicentre collaborative approach is more likely than single-centre studies to gen-

80

erate significant epidemiological and clinical knowledge. Several multicentre collaborative groups are now in existence, for example the Canadian Collaborative Study Group, which consists of 14 regionally based MS clinics across Canada with approximately 15 000 well-characterized patients followed prospectively over a long period of time. Many of these clinics have adopted a common database called MS COSTAR, which can be used to pool data from the various Canadian clinics. In recent years, this group has produced considerable information on genetic susceptibility to MS, derived from studies that have included twin concordance rates (Sadovnick et al., 1993) and risk in adoptees (Ebers, Sadovnick & Risch, 1995). Other such groups have been formed in Europe, and 20 centres across participating countries have combined to form the European Concerted Action on MS, which has adopted a common database known as EDMUS. Two of their major collaborations to date are a prospective study on the effects of pregnancy in MS (Hours et al., 1995) and another on clinical and paraclinical features that may predict MS outcome (Moreau et al., 1995).

Multicentre databases could also be used to identify sufficient patients in either high- or low-risk groups to allow the study of possible environmental risk factors. For example, twins and biological relatives of MS patients have a higher risk of MS, providing an intrinsic correction for genetic susceptibility; case–control studies that compared the environments of relatives who do or do not develop MS might therefore be most instructive. Although some research on risk factors in twins has been conducted (Currier & Eldridge, 1982), more is needed. Since MS is very uncommon in some racial or ethnic groups, such as the Japanese and the Hutterites, studies that matched MS cases from resistant groups with controls from the same racial or ethnic background might provide significant clues to etiology.

5.3 Factors associated with acquisition versus clinical manifestation

Evidence suggests that factors influencing the acquisition of MS may differ from those that play a role in determining clinical manifestation. For example, Europeans who migrate to South Africa before the age of 15 experience a greater reduction in MS risk than older immigrants (Dean & Kurtzke, 1971), presumably because they have had less time to acquire some causal factor that is more common (or more likely to be acquired) in their homeland. Older immigrants do experience some reduction in risk, however, which indicates that, although more of them may have acquired a causal factor in their homeland, a protective factor in their new country operates against onset of the disease—otherwise their risk should be the same as it would be in their country of origin.

Failure to recognize the possibility that acquisition and clinical manifestation of disease may be influenced by entirely different factors could mask the effects of exposures specific to each. Case–control studies that have simply measured exposure before disease onset—despite evidence from migrant studies that an important environmental cause operates in early adolescence—can be used to illustrate this problem. The extended data collection period will obviously include the etiologically important exposure but may also incorporate years of irrelevant exposure, leading to potential misclassification of patients and controls. For example, exposure to dogs may be associated with acquisition but not with onset. If patients and controls were asked specifically about exposure to dogs before the age of 15, they might report a difference. If, however, more controls than patients were for some reason exposed to dogs after age 15, there might be no difference between the groups in response to questions about exposure at any time before onset age. Risk-factor studies should be designed to take account of this possibility.

5.4 Narrowing windows of exposure

Since onset of MS peaks around age 30, using the age of 15 as the dividing point for the pre-onset age period still leaves wide intervals of exposure. Researchers have had some success in narrowing the "window" period of acquisition through migration studies and modelling based on the apparent latent period between acquisition and onset, but less effort has been devoted to narrowing the "window" of onset.

Migrant studies indicate that at least one important environmental risk factor operates before age 15. The number of immigrants under age 15 is generally too small to allow any meaningful age-stratification to narrow the timing of exposure. From available migration data, however, Kurtzke (1972) suggested that acquisition is concentrated between 12 and 15 years of age and that, since peak onset is around age 30, the latency period in MS is close to 20 years. Geographical cluster studies that have found evidence of pre-onset age clustering among patients (Eastman, Sheridan & Poskanzer, 1973; Poskanzer et al., 1981) also support a 20-year latency period but have not been specifically used to narrow the timing of exposure beyond about age 15. Wolfson, Wolfson & Zielinski (1989) have constructed a model for the pre-onset age natural history of MS and used it to estimate the distribution of the latent period of the disease. All patients in their study were assumed to have acquired MS over a fixed susceptibility period. Their approach allowed them to consider several such periods: 0–5, 0–10, 0–15, 5–15, and 10–15 years. They deduced that the most likely window of exposure was 10–15 years of age and estimated average latency as 18–19 years. Considering the results of migration and modelling studies that have attempted to define a typical acquisition period, questions about exposure in case–control studies should probably be concentrated between the ages of 10 and 15.

Narrowing the window of relevant onset-related exposure seems more complex because the induction period (that is, the time from an acquisition-related exposure to disease initiation) is unknown. The latency period in MS is generally defined as the interval from acquisition (that is, around age 15) to onset. However, this definition is based on the assumption that disease initiation is close to acquisition, since the formal definition of latent period is the time from disease initiation until a patient or physician first detects symptoms. In reality, while initiation may be close to acquisition, there is evidence to suggest that it should not necessarily be equated with onset. Autopsies in asymptomatic patients have revealed lesions that, based on their location, would have been especially likely to give rise to abnormal signs (Namerow & Thompson, 1969; Ghatak et al., 1974). There may be several possible explanations: these individuals may not have been exposed to an enhancing factor associated with clinical manifestation or were insufficiently exposed; alternatively, they may have been exposed to some factor that protected them against onset. Nevertheless, this observation suggests not only the importance of onset-related exposures but also that the interval from initiation to onset may be variable, or even infinite, rather than brief. Geographical cluster studies may provide some insight into this time period, since Poskanzer et al. (1981) observed two temporal–spatial clusterings of patients on the Orkney Islands—the first about 21 years before onset, and a second just before onset—which may have represented common exposure to an onset-related factor. On the other hand, Riise et al. (1991) observed peak geographical clustering of patients around age 18 in a Norwegian birth cohort. Since this cluster is beyond the generally accepted acquisition window, it might represent an onset-related exposure and would indicate a longer period from exposure to onset than is suggested by the data of Poskanzer et al. Variability in the window of exposure to onset-related factors might indicate a cumulative process influenced by environmental intensity.

5.5 Retrospective versus prospective studies

Because the interval from acquisition to onset is so long and many patients interviewed in retrospective studies are well beyond onset, participants' early adolescence may be 20–50 years in the past. Only the most concrete, relatively long-term exposures related to acquisition, such as living on a farm, are likely to be reported accurately by either patients or controls. Variables such as exposure to infectious diseases or diet may be impossible to assess.

There are several approaches to dealing with recall. One would be to include only early-onset patients and interview them as soon after diagnosis as possible. Since onset before the age of 20 is relatively rare (typically less than 20%), multicentre collaboration would be necessary to identify sufficient cases. Newly diagnosed patients may be preoccupied with adjusting to the disease and unwilling to participate in epidemiological studies, so that the importance of their cooperation would have to be stressed. Verification of information by available family physicians, parents, and siblings is not likely to be useful since their recall of the experiences of patients and controls may also be inaccurate. Written records may not have been kept or may prove to be incomplete.

The introduction of universal medical coverage in some countries and computerization of data on use of health care services have made prospective risk factor studies in MS possible. In the Canadian province of Alberta, for example, Svenson (1996, personal communication) is following a cohort of several thousand children. Provided that there is an etiological factor (such as an infectious disease) for which children are typically treated by a physician, it might be possible to detect differences between children who develop MS later and those who do not. Prospective studies would help to avoid not only inaccurate recall but also recall bias. However, this approach is obviously limited by the information collected, its accuracy, and its completeness.

Research into onset-related factors in retrospective studies may also experience problems associated with recall. Although exposure to these factors will have been more recent than acquisition-related exposures, it is still likely to have occurred in the relatively distant past. Relapses might be examined as proxies for onset-related exposures since factors that precipitate onset may well be similar to factors that precipitate subsequent relapses. Although relapses are more recent than disease onset, the interval of time before relapse about which patients should be questioned is unclear—and recall is probably less reliable the longer the interval. Moreover, patients in relapse may also be biased in their recall of recent events if they associate a particular factor with exacerbation. It may be possible to avoid these problems in prospective relapse studies, for example by asking patients to keep diaries of events or behaviours between relapses. However, prospective studies based on clinical manifestation will not distinguish between factors related to disease activity and those related to overt relapse, since research indicates that exacerbations may have been building for some time before symptoms occur (Matthews, 1985). Techniques such as MRI are able to track changes in disease activity (for example, a decrease in plaque size) as illustrated in Fig. 6, regardless of symptoms. An MRI can be remarkably abnormal, with multiple plaques in the brain and spinal cord, without the patient showing any signs of the disease. Using MRI, it has been shown that relapses may occur in clinically silent areas of the brain while the patient experiences no clinical features. Future epidemiological studies should be linked more closely to MRI testing and/or CSF immunochemistry studies. However, the use of such expensive techniques in prospective studies of factors related to clinical manifestation may not be generally feasible.

5.6 Possible different forms of multiple sclerosis

Most case–control studies of MS have grouped all patients together and examined overall risk factors. However, the clinical variability of the disease has led researchers to suggest that MS consists of two or more diseases (Cazzullo et al., 1978; Detels et al., 1982; Poser, Raun & Poser, 1982; Noseworthy et al., 1983; Lyon-Caen et al., 1985; Izquierdo et al., 1986; Larsen et al., 1986; Van Lambalgen, Sanders & D'Amaro, 1986; Duquette et al., 1987). "Early onset" MS is more common among women, tends to present with ON or sensory symptoms, and is more likely to follow an RR or benign course. Conversely, "late onset" MS is more common among men and tends to present with motor disturbances and to follow a CP or disabling course.

***Fig. 6. Magnetic resonance imaging of the brain of a patient with multiple
sclerosis***
A dramatic number of inflammatory–demyelinating lesions can be seen in
the periventricular and subcortical white matter of both cerebral hemispheres, extending from the frontal lobes anteriorly to the parietal–occip-
ital lobes posteriorly (top left). The differential diagnosis of this 22-year-old
female patient included multiple sclerosis and post-infectious encephalomyelitis. A repeat MRI of the brain 6 months later illustrates resolu-
tion of the MS plaques (top right). A further MRI 3 years later, when the
patient was in clinical remission, illustrates small residual lesions in the
centrum ovale (bottom)

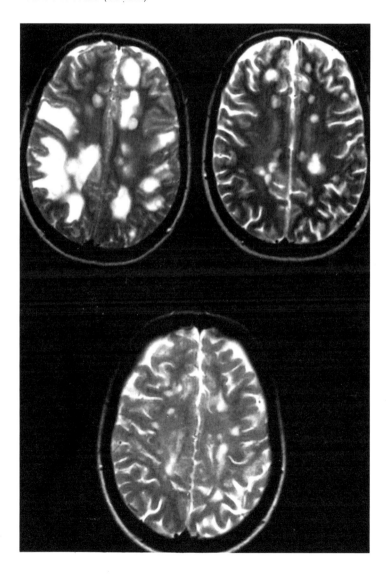

There are examples of other diseases that exist in more than one form, such as diabetes mellitus (insulin-dependent and non-insulin-dependent), and with somewhat different etiologies. If there are indeed two forms of MS, the practice of grouping all patients together in case–control studies may mask the effect of risk factors associated with either form.

Fischman (1982) suggested that risk factors may differ according to age of onset, since there is descriptive evidence that onset age varies with urban/rural residence (Alter, 1962; Poskanzer, Schapira & Miller, 1963a; Detels et al., 1978; Roberts, 1986) and ethnicity (Dean & Kurtzke, 1971; Acheson, 1985). However, it seems that only one analytical study has examined whether risk factors vary with onset age. Dividing MS patients into early-, intermediate-, and late-onset age groups, Warren, Cockerill & Warren (1991) compared the groups with each other on personal and disease characteristics and with healthy controls on risk factors related to residence and family background (including ethnicity). There were no statistically significant differences between the onset-age groups in sex, presenting symptoms, or disability, although trends followed the expected direction. Four risk factors distinguished between patients and controls overall, namely rural residence, use of well water, and family histories of MS and of diabetes. The only factor that showed a definite link with onset age was a family history of diabetes, which was more important for early onset. By contrast, use of well water was apparently more important for intermediate to late onset. Small sample sizes, especially in the early- and late-onset categories may have interfered with the detection of significant differences. However, to the extent that differences did exist, this study suggests that host susceptibility factors may predispose to early onset, whereas environmental factors may play a more important role in intermediate- to late-onset MS.

Warren et al. (1993a) have also examined risk factors by sex. Data were collected from MS patients on personal and disease characteristics; both patients and controls were questioned about infectious disease history, family history of illness, and ethnicity, because it has been suggested (Van Lambalgen, Sanders & D'Amaro, 1986) that an infectious disease trigger is more important in men and susceptibility more important in women. Although male and female patients did not differ in age at onset, presenting symptoms, or disability, trends were in the expected direction. The only risk factor that differed between male patients and controls was MS family history. This factor also differed between female patients and controls, as did herpes labialis infection, later age of mumps, a family history of diabetes, and northern European ancestry of both parents. Some of these factors also distinguished between patients as a whole and controls, but none showed evidence of interaction with sex. The findings of this study do not support the theory that an infectious disease trigger is more important in men, but the small number of men may have precluded detection of significant differences. Considering the preponderance of female MS patients, this study might be worth repeating with a larger number of males and including other potential risk factors such as those related to occupation.

No studies published to date appear to have grouped patients by presenting symptoms or by primary RR versus CP disease course. Alternatively, risk factors could be compared by sporadic versus familial MS. Weinshenker et al. (1990) have suggested that any etiological heterogeneity would manifest itself primarily in differences between patients with a family history of MS and those without: presumably, environmental triggers would be more important for sporadic cases and genetic susceptibility for familial MS. Before examining risk factors, these researchers opted to compare personal and disease characteristics of patients with sporadic MS with those of patients with familial MS, to determine whether they appear to represent two forms of MS. There were no differences between sporadic and familial cases in age at onset, sex, presenting symptom, disease course (whether primary RR or CP), occurrence of acute relapse at onset, number of attacks in the first 2 years, or interval between first and second attack. When familial cases were grouped according to the number of other relatives with MS and degree of the relationship, there was some variability between groups in sex, whether disease was primary RR or CP, and rate of progression to a given disability level. Warren et al. (1993b) have confirmed the absence of differences in clinical features between familial and sporadic MS. They also collected data from patients and matched controls on: urban/rural residence and related factors, infectious disease history, and family background (including ethnicity, socioeconomic status and history of illness). The only variable to differ between patients and controls overall and to show evidence of interaction with familial versus sporadic MS was the mother's ethnicity—patients with familial MS were more likely to have a mother with northern European, rather than British, ancestry.

Finally, for the purpose of risk factor studies, patients might be grouped according to the immunological form of their disease. Although there may be several, Warren et al. (1994) have identified at least two immunologically distinct forms of MS: anti-myelin basic protein (anti-MBP) associated MS and anti-proteolipid protein (anti-PLP) associated MS. Warren & Warren (1995) compared various personal and disease characteristics of patients with anti-MBP and anti-PLP disease. They found that significantly more anti-PLP patients were male and experienced onset after age 40, whereas significantly more anti-MBP patients had a family history of MS. There were no obvious differences in presenting symptoms, and the majority of patients in both groups were ambulatory, although average illness duration was insufficient to allow speculation about eventual disability. The differences that did exist may indicate etiological heterogeneity.

5.7 Prenatal risk factors

The possibility of prenatal risk factors has received scant attention in MS epidemiology. Research has indicated that some prenatal factor might be involved in the etiology of schizophrenia—an illness with a north–south gradient similar to MS (Torrey, 1987)—because there appears to be an excess of late winter or spring births among treated schizophrenics. Speculation has revolved primarily around a viral infection in pregnant women since exposure to infections might vary by season of gestation. Researchers have looked for an association between the incidence of births of schizophrenic patients and the incidence of various infections in the previous 12 months, broken down by trimester of exposure. They have also examined whether mothers of children who developed schizophrenia were pregnant during a recorded viral epidemic, whether their medical records revealed treatment for any viral infection, and whether they had young children who could have introduced infection into the home during the pregnancy. There are several biologically plausible explanations for such a hypothesis. For example, exposure to a virus could interfere with cell migration in the fetal brain and produce a post-infectious encephalitis with a latency of 15 years or more. Alternatively, a virus could predispose to later development of an autoimmune disease (Torrey, Rawlings & Waldman, 1988). It is also possible that some unidentified infectious agent, with a periodicity similar to the viral infection, is responsible, or that drugs used by the mother to combat the infection produced an effect on the fetus (Beiser & Iacono, 1990).

Diseases that share a similar distribution may also share etiological risk factors. It might therefore be worth examining season of birth of MS patients and prenatal exposure to viral infections, much as these factors have been examined in schizophrenia patients. There are other avenues that might also be explored. For example, a viral hypothesis predicts that the association with season of birth would be stronger in sporadic than familial MS cases. Moreover, if variation with the season of birth is the result of a neurodevelopmental effect, the birth date should be associated with different onset age, course, and outcome of MS. This type of study, which has proved valuable in schizophrenia, might help to uncover a risk factor that is important in a significant percentage of MS patients.

5.8 Final note

Weinshenker (1995) has summarized the ideal conditions that should exist for epidemiological research to reveal an environmental cause:

- The population being studied is highly susceptible to the disease.
- Individuals within that population are uniformly susceptible.
- The disease is distinctive, with no phenocopies or subclinical forms.
- The causal factor has a high attack rate with a short incubation period.
- The disease is acquired through a single mechanism.

- The biological mechanism of interaction between the environmental cause and the host is understood.

At the same time, Weinshenker points out that MS violates most, if not all, of these conditions. Nevertheless, epidemiological research has already contributed important clues to the etiology of the disease. As remaining methodological issues are resolved, the opportunities for epidemiology to make additional contributions will increase.

References

Achari AN, Trontelj JV, Campos DJ (1976). Multiple sclerosis and myasthenia gravis. A case report with single fiber electromyography. *Neurology*, 26:544–546.

Acheson ED (1961). Multiple sclerosis in British Commonwealth countries in the southern hemisphere. *British Journal of Preventive Social Medicine*, 15:118–125.

Acheson ED (1985). The epidemiology of multiple sclerosis: the pattern of the disease. In: Matthews WB, ed. *McAlpine's multiple sclerosis*. Edinburgh, Churchill Livingstone: Chapter 1.

Acheson ED, Bachrach C, Wright F (1960). Some comments on the relationship of the distribution of multiple sclerosis to latitude, solar radiation and other variables. *Acta Psychiatrica Scandinavica*, 35(Suppl. 147):132–147.

Ackerman A (1931). Die multiple sklerose in der Schweiz. [Multiple sclerosis in Switzerland.] *Schweizerische Medizinische Wochenschrift*, 61:1245–1250.

Adam A (1989). Multiple sclerosis: epidemic in Kenya. *East African Medical Journal*, 66:503–506.

Afoke AO et al. (1993). Seasonal variation and sex differences of circulating macrophages, immunoglobulins and lymphocytes in healthy school children. *Scandinavian Journal of Immunology*, 37:209–215.

Agranoff BWA, Goldberg D (1974). Diet and the geographical distribution of multiple sclerosis. *Lancet*, ii:1061–1066.

Aita JF, Snyder DH, Reichl W (1974). Myasthenia gravis and multiple sclerosis: an unusual combination of diseases. *Neurology*, 24:72–75.

Ajdacic-Gross V (1994). The male sex is more subject to disseminated sclerosis than the female. In: *Multiple sclerosis epidemiology: analytical approaches to the study of etiology. Abstracts from the Oslo International Think-tank on Multiple Sclerosis Epidemiology, Centre for Advanced Studies, Oslo, September 17–18, 1994*. Copenhagen, Munksgaard:12.

Alaev B (1994). The epidemiology of multiple sclerosis in Uzbekistan. In: Firnhaber W, Lauer K, eds. *Multiple sclerosis in Europe: an epidemiological update*. Darmstadt, LTV Press:236–240.

Al-Din AS (1986). Multiple sclerosis in Kuwait: clinical and epidemiological study. *Journal of Neurology, Neurosurgery and Psychiatry*, 49:928–931.

Al-Din AS et al. (1991). Epidemiology of multiple sclerosis in Kuwait: a comparative study between Kuwaitis and Palestinians. *Journal of Neurological Sciences*, 100:137–141.

Allison RS, Millar JHD (1954). Prevalence and familial incidence of disseminated sclerosis (a report to the Northern Ireland Hospitals Authority on the results of a three-year study). Prevalence of disseminated sclerosis in Northern Ireland. *Ulster Medical Journal*, 23(Suppl. 2):5–92.

Alpérovitch A, Bouvier MH (1982). Geographical pattern of death rates from multiple sclerosis in France. An analysis of 4912 deaths. *Acta Neurologica Scandinavica*, 66:454–461.

Alter M (1962). Multiple sclerosis in the negro. *Archives of Neurology*, 7:83–91.

Alter M, Cendrowski W (1976). Multiple sclerosis and childhood infections. *Neurology*, 26:201–204.

Alter M, Speer J (1968). Clinical evaluation of possible etiologic factors in multiple sclerosis. *Neurology*, 18:109–116.

Alter M, Leibowitz U, Speer J (1966). Risk of multiple sclerosis related to age at immigration to Israel. *Archives of Neurology*, 15:234–237.

Alter M, Yamoor M, Harshe M (1974). Multiple sclerosis and nutrition. *Archives of Neurology*, 31:267–272.

Alter M et al. (1960). Geographic distribution of multiple sclerosis. A comparison of prevalence in Charleston County, South Carolina, USA, and Halifax County, Nova Scotia, Canada. *World Neurology*, 1:55–70.

Alter M et al. (1968). Epidemiology of multiple sclerosis in Israel. In: Alter M, Kurtzke J, eds. *The epidemiology of multiple sclerosis*. Springfield, IL, Charles C. Thomas:83–109.

Alter M et al. (1971). MS among Orientals and Caucasians in Hawaii. *Neurology*, 21:122–130.

Alter M et al. (1986). Multiple sclerosis and childhood infections. *Neurology*, 36:1386–1389.

Alvord EC Jr et al. (1987). The multiple cases of multiple sclerosis: the importance of infections in childhood. *Journal of Child Neurology*, 2:313–321.

Amato MP et al. (1999). A prospective study on the natural history of multiple sclerosis: clues to the conduct and interpretation of clinical trials. *Journal of the Neurological Sciences*, 168:96–106.

Amprino D et al. (1977). Ricerca epidemiologica sulla sclerosi multipla nella provincia di Bari. [Research on the epidemiology of multiple sclerosis in the province of Bari.] *Acta Neurologica (Napoli)*, 32:818–832.]

Anderson DW et al. (1992). Revised estimate of the prevalence of multiple sclerosis in the United States. *Annals of Neurology*, 31:333–336.

Anderson LJ et al. (1984). Multiple sclerosis unrelated to dog exposure. *Neurology*, 34:1149–1154.

Andersson M et al. (1994). The role of cerebrospinal fluid analysis in the diagnosis of multiple sclerosis: a consensus report. *Journal of Neurology, Neurosurgery and Psychiatry*, 57:897–902.

Angeleri F et al. (1989). A prevalence study of multiple sclerosis in the Regione Marche, Italy. In: Battaglia MA, Crimi G, eds. *An update on multiple sclerosis*. Bologna, Monduzzi Editore:209–212.

Antonovsky A et al. (1968). Reappraisal of possible etiological factors in multiple sclerosis. *American Journal of Public Health and the Nation's Health*, 58:836–848.

Baldwin A (1952). Case of disseminated sclerosis following injury. *West London Medical Journal*, 12:214.

Bamford CR et al. (1981). Trauma as an etiologic and aggravating factor in multiple sclerosis. *Neurology*, 31:1229–1234.

Barlow J (1960). Correlation of the geographic distribution of multiple sclerosis with cosmic ray intensities. *Acta Neurological Scandinavica*, 35(S147):108–130.

Barton DE, David FN, Merrington M (1965). A criterion for testing congregation in space and time. *Annals of Human Genetics*, 29:97–102.

Bartschi-Rochaix W (1980). MS in Switzerland Canton Wallis. In: Bauer H et al., eds. *Progress in multiple sclerosis research*. New York, Springer:535–538.

Batchelor JR (1985). Immunological and genetic aspects of multiple sclerosis. In: Matthews WB, ed. *McAlpine's multiple sclerosis*. Edinburgh, Churchill Livingstone: Chapter 11.

Bates D (1993). The diagnosis of multiple sclerosis. In: *Proceedings of the MS Forum Modern Management Workshop*. Worthington, England, Professional Postgraduate Services Europe: Chapter 4.

Bauer HJ (1980). IMAB-enquête concerning the diagnostic criteria for multiple sclerosis. In: Bauer HJ et al., eds. *Progress in multiple sclerosis*. Berlin, Springer:555–563.

Bauer HJ (1987). Multiple sclerosis in Europe. *Journal of Neurology*, 234:195–206.

Bauer HJ, Wikström J (1978). Multiple sclerosis and house pets. *Lancet*, 2:1029.

Beebe GW et al. (1967). Studies on the natural history of multiple sclerosis. 3. Epidemiologic analysis of the army experience in World War II. *Neurology*, 17:1–17.

Beer S, Kesselring J (1994). High prevalence of multiple sclerosis in Switzerland. *Neuroepidemiology*, 13:14–18.

Behrend R (1966). Prevalence of multiple sclerosis in Hamburg and Marseille. *Acta Neurologica Scandinavica*, 42(Suppl. 19):27–42.

Behrend R et al. (1963). Etude statistique sur la sclérose en plaques à Marseille. [Statistical study of multiple sclerosis in Marseilles.] *Revue Neurologique*, 109:630–634.

Beiser M, Iacono WG (1990). An update on the epidemiology of schizophrenia. *Canadian Journal of Psychiatry*, 35:657–668.

Ben Hamida M (1977). La sclérose en plaques en Tunisie: étude clinique de 100 observations. [Multiple sclerosis in Tunisia: clinical study with 100 cases.] *Revue Neurologique*, 33:109–117.

Bencsik K et al. (1998). The prevalence of multiple sclerosis in the Hungarian city of Szeged. *Acta Neurologica Scandinavica*, 97:315–319.

Benedikz JEG (1994). The natural history of multiple sclerosis in Iceland. A total population study. In: *Multiple sclerosis epidemiology: analytical approaches to the study of etiology. Abstracts from the Oslo International Think-tank on Multiple Sclerosis Epidemiology, Centre for Advanced Study, Oslo, September 17–18, 1994.* Copenhagen, Munskgaard:37.

Benedikz J et al. (1994). Multiple sclerosis in Iceland. 1 January 1980–31 December 1989: a 9 year total population study. In: Firnhaber W, Lauder K, eds. *Multiple sclerosis in Europe: an epidemiological update.* Darmstadt, LTV Press:41–50.

Benedikz J, Magnusson H, Guthmundsson G (1994). Multiple sclerosis in Iceland; with observations on the alleged epidemic in the Faroe Islands. *Annals of Neurology*, 36(Suppl. 2):S175–S179.

Bennett L et al. (1977). Survey of persons with multiple sclerosis in Ottawa, 1974–1975. *Canadian Journal of Public Health*, 68:141–147.

Berr C et al. (1989). Risk-factors in multiple sclerosis: a population-based case-control study in Hautes-Pyrénées, France. *Acta Neurologica Scandinavica*, 80:46–50.

Binzer M et al. (1994). Familial clustering of multiple sclerosis in a northern Swedish rural district. *Journal of Neurology, Neurosurgery and Psychiatry*, 57:497–499.

Biton V, Abramsky V (1986). Newer study fails to support environmental factor in etiology of MS. *Neurology*, 36(S1):184.

Bixenman WW, Buchsbaum HW (1988). Multiple sclerosis, euthyroid restrictive Graves' ophthalmology, and myasthenia gravis: a case report. *Graefes Archive for Clinical and Experimental Ophthalmology*, 226:168–171.

Bobowick A et al. (1978). Twin study of multiple sclerosis: an epidemiologic inquiry. *Neurology*, 28:978–987.

Boiko AN (1994). Multiple sclerosis prevalence in Russia and other countries of the former USSR. In: Firnhaber W, Lauer K, eds. *Multiple sclerosis in Europe: an epidemiological update.* Darmstadt, LTV Press:219–230.

Boiko A et al. (1995). Epidemiology of multiple sclerosis in Russia and other countries of the former Soviet Union: investigations of environmental and genetic factors. *Acta Neurologica Scandinavica Supplementum*, 161:71–76.

Bourneville DM (1892). *Oeuvres complètes de JM Charcot: leçons sur les maladies du système nerveux, Vol. 1. [The complete works of JM Charcot: lessons on conditions of the nervous system.]* Paris, Félix Alcan:189–272.

Braceland FJ, Giffin ME (1950). The mental changes associated with multiple sclerosis. *Proceedings of the Association for Research on Nervous and Mental Diseases*, 28:450–455.

Brain WR (1930). Critical review: disseminated sclerosis. *Quarterly Journal of Medicine*, 23:343–391.

Brassat D et al. (1999). Familial factors influence disability in MS multiplex families. French Multiple Sclerosis Genetics Group. *Neurology*, 52:1632–1636.

Breslow NE, Day NE (1988). *Statistical methods in cancer research. Vol. 2: The design and analysis of cohort studies.* New York, Oxford University Press:48–79.

Brody JA (1972). Epidemiology of multiple sclerosis and a possible virus aetiology. *Lancet*, ii:173–176.

Bufill E et al. (1995). Prevalence of multiple sclerosis in the region of Osona, Catalonia, northern Spain. *Journal of Neurology, Neurosurgery and Psychiatry*, 58:577–581.

Bulman D, Ebers G (1992). The geography of MS reflects genetic susceptibility. *Journal of Tropical and Geographical Neurology*, 2:66–72.

Bulman DE et al. (1991). Age of onset in siblings concordant for multiple sclerosis. *Brain*, 114:937–950.

Bunnell DH, Visscher BR, Detels R (1979). Multiple sclerosis and housedogs: a case-control study. *Neurology*, 29:1027–1029.

Butcher PJ (1992). Calcium intake and the protein composition of mouse brain: relevance to multiple sclerosis. *Medical Hypotheses*, 39:275–280.

Callegaro D et al. (1992). Prevalence of multiple sclerosis in the city of Sao Paulo, Brazil, in 1990. *Neuroepidemiology*, 11:11–14.

Campbell AMG et al. (1947). Disease of the nervous system occurring among research workers on swayback in lambs. *Brain*, 70:50–58.

Canadian Burden of Illness Study Group (1998). Burden of illness of multiple sclerosis: part I: cost of illness. *Canadian Journal of Neurological Sciences*, 25:23–30.

Cantorna MT (2000). Vitamin D and autoimmunity: is vitamin D status an environmental factor affecting autoimmune disease prevalence? *Proceedings of the Society for Experimental Biology and Medicine*, 223:230–233.

Caputo D et al. (1979). Epidemiological study of multiple sclerosis in the province of Novara. *Acta Neurologica (Napoli)*, 1:133–141.

Casetta I et al. (1998). An epidemiological study of multiple sclerosis in central Sardinia, Italy. *Acta Neurologica Scandinavica*, 98:391–394.

Cazzullo CL et al. (1973). Studio epidemiologico della sclerosi multipla: esemplo di ricerca epidemiologica in neurologia. [Epidemiological study of multiple sclerosis: an example of epidemiological research in neurology.] *Riversta Neurobiologica (Napoli)*, 19:165–174.

Cazzullo CL et al. (1978). Clinical picture of multiple sclerosis with late onset. *Acta Neurologica Scandinavica*, 58:190–196.

Cendrowski W (1966). An unusual cluster of cases of multiple sclerosis in northern Poland. *Journal of the Neurological Sciences*, 3:349–352.

Cendrowski W et al. (1969). Epidemiological study of multiple sclerosis in western Poland. *European Neurology*, 2:90–108.

Cernacek J et al. (1971). The relation of geographical and meteorological factors to the occurrence of multiple sclerosis in Czechoslovakia. *Acta Neurologica Scandinavica*, 47:227–232.

Chan WW (1977). Multiple sclerosis and dogs. *Lancet*, i:487–488.

Chandra V et al. (1984). Mortality data for the US for deaths due to and related to twenty neurologic diseases. *Neuroepidemiology*, 3:149–168.

Charcot JM (1868). Histologie de la sclérose en plaques. [Histology of multiple sclerosis.] *Gazette Hôpital Paris*, 41:554–555.

Chataway J et al. (1998). The genetics of multiple sclerosis: principles, background and updated results of the United Kingdom genome screen. *Brain*, 121:1869–1887.

Chipman M (1966). Multiple sclerosis in Houston, Texas, 1954–1959. A study of the methodology used in determining the prevalence in a large southern city. *Acta Neurologica Scandinavica*, 42(Suppl. 19):77–82.

Compston A (1990). Risk factors for multiple sclerosis: race or place? *Journal of Neurology, Neurosurgery and Psychiatry*, 53:821–823.

Compston DAS (1999). The genetic epidemiology of multiple sclerosis. *Philosophical Transactions of the Royal Society of London. Series B: Biological Sciences*, 354:1623–1634.

Compston DAS et al. (1995). Genes and susceptibility to multiple sclerosis. *Acta Neurologica Scandinavica Supplementum*, 161:43–51.

Confavreux C et al. (1987). Le sud-est français, zone à haute risque de sclérose en plaques? [South-east France, a high-risk zone for multiple sclerosis?] *Presse médicale*, 16:622: 623.

Cook SD, Dowling PC (1977). A possible association between house pets and multiple sclerosis. *Lancet*, i:980–982.

Cook SD, Dowling PC (1981). Distemper and multiple sclerosis in Sitka, Alaska. *Annals of Neurology*, 11:192–194.

Cook SD, Dowling PC, Russell WC (1978). Multiple sclerosis and canine distemper. *Lancet*, i:605–606.

Cook SD et al. (1978). Further evidence of a possible association between house dogs and multiple sclerosis. *Annals of Neurology*, 3:141–143.

Cook SD et al. (1985). Declining evidence of multiple sclerosis in the Orkney islands. *Neurology*, 35:545–551.

Cook SD et al. (1988). Multiple sclerosis in the Shetland Islands: an update. *Acta Neurologica Scandinavica*, 77:148–151.

Cook SD et al. (1995). Evidence for multiple sclerosis as an infectious disease. *Acta Neurologica Scandinavica Supplementum*, 161:34–42.

Craelius W (1978). Comparative epidemiology of multiple sclerosis and dental caries. *Journal of Epidemiology and Community Health*, 32:155–165.

Cunningham J (1972). The prevalence of multiple sclerosis in Christchurch. *New Zealand Medical Journal*, 76:417–418.

Currier RD, Eldridge R (1982). Possible risk factors in multiple sclerosis as found in a national twin study. *Archives of Neurology*, 39:140–144.

Currier RD, Martin EA, Woosley PC (1974). Prior events in multiple sclerosis. *Neurology*, 24:748–754.

Curtius F (1933). *Multiple sklerose und Erbanlage. [Multiple sclerosis and heredity.]* Leipzig, Thieme.

Dalos NP et al. (1983). Disease activity and emotional state in multiple sclerosis. *Annals of Neurology*, 13:573–577.

Dassel H (1972). Discussion of the epidemiology of MS. In: Field EJ, Bell TM, Carnegie PR, eds. *Multiple sclerosis: progress in research*. Amsterdam, North-Holland:241–242.

D'Aurizio C et al. (1988). Prevalenza della sclerosi multipla nel commune di L'Aquila, Italia centrale. [Prevalence of multiple sclerosis in the community of l'Aquila, central Italy.] In: Cosi V, Citterio A, eds. *V Convegno Nazionale di Neuroepidemiologia. [Fifth Nation Congress on Neuroepidemiology.]* Pavia, La Goliardica Pavese:133–136.

Davenport C (1922). Multiple sclerosis: from the standpoint of geographic distribution and race. *Archives of Neurology and Psychiatry*, 8:51–58.

Dean G (1967). Annual incidence, prevalence, and mortality of multiple sclerosis in white South-African-born and in white immigrants to South Africa. *British Medical Journal*, 2:724–730.

Dean G, Kurtzke J (1971). On the risk of multiple sclerosis according to age at immigration to South Africa. *British Medical Journal*, 3:725–729.

Dean G, Goodall J, Downie A (1981). The prevalence of multiple sclerosis in the Outer Hebrides compared with north-east Scotland and the Orkney and Shetland Islands. *Journal of Epidemiology and Community Health*, 35:110–113.

Dean G et al. (1976). Multiple sclerosis among immigrants in Greater London. *British Medical Journal*, 1:861–864.

Dean G et al. (1977). Motor neurone disease and multiple sclerosis among immigrants to Britain. *British Journal of Preventive and Social Medicine*, 31:141–147.

Dean G et al. (1979). Multiple sclerosis in southern Europe. I: Prevalence in Sicily in 1975. *Journal of Epidemiology and Community Health*, 33:107–110.

Dean G et al. (1981). The prevalence of multiple sclerosis in Sicily. I: Agrigento city. *Journal of Epidemiology and Community Health*, 35:118–122.

Detels R et al. (1977). Evidence for lower susceptibility to multiple sclerosis among Japanese-Americans. *American Journal of Epidemiology*, 105:303–310.

Detels R et al. (1978). Multiple sclerosis and age at migration. *American Journal of Epidemiology*, 108:386–393.

Detels R et al. (1982). Factors associated with a rapid course of multiple sclerosis. *Archives of Neurology*, 39:337–341.

Diabetes Epidemiology Research International Group (1988). Geographic patterns of childhood insulin-dependent diabetes mellitus. *Diabetes*, 37:1113–1119.

Diodato S et al. (1989). Multiple sclerosis epidemiological survey in Pordenone. In: Battaglia MA, Crimi G, eds. *An update on multiple sclerosis*. Bologna, Monduzzi Editore:231–233.

Dubos R (1965). *Man adapting*. New Haven, CT, Yale University Press.

Duquette P et al. (1987). Multiple sclerosis in childhood: clinical profile in 125 patients. *Journal of Pediatrics*, 111:359–363.

Eastman R, Sheridan J, Poskanzer DC (1973). Multiple sclerosis clustering in a small Massachusetts community with possible common exposure 23 years before onset. *New England Journal of Medicine*, 289:793–794.

Ebers G, Sadovnick AD, Risch NJ (1995). A genetic basis for familial aggregation in multiple sclerosis. Canadian Collaborative Study Group. *Nature*, 377:150–151.

Ederer F, Myers MH, Mantel N (1964). A statistical problem in space and time: do leukemia cases come in clusters? *Biometrics*, 20:626–638.

Edgely KM, Sullivan JL, Dehoux E (1991). A survey of multiple sclerosis. Part II: Determinants of employment status. *Canadian Journal of Rehabilitation*, 4:127–132.

Eichorst H (1913). Multiple sklerose und spastische spinal paralyse. [Multiple sclerosis and spastic spinal paralysis.] *Medizinische Klinik*, 9:1617–1619.

Eldridge R et al. (1978). Familial multiple sclerosis: clinical, histocompatibility and viral serological studies. *Annals of Neurology*, 3:72–80.

Elian M, Nightingale S, Dean G (1990). Multiple sclerosis among the United Kingdom-born children of immigrants from the Indian subcontinent, Africa and the West Indies. *Journal of Neurology, Neurosurgery and Psychiatry*, 53:906–911.

Esberg S, Keiding N, Koch-Henriksen N (1999). Reporting delay and corrected incidence of multiple sclerosis. *Statistics in Medicine*, 18:1691–1706.

Esparza ML, Sasaki S, Kesteloot H (1995). Nutrition, latitude and multiple sclerosis: an ecologic study. *American Journal of Epidemiology*, 142:733–737.

Fernandez O, Bufill E (1994). Prevalence of multiple sclerosis in Spain: validation of an epidemiological protocol in two geographically separated areas. In: Firnhaber W, Lauer K, eds. *Multiple sclerosis in Europe: an epidemiological update*. Darmstadt, LTV Press:184–189.

Firth D (1948). *The case of Augustus d'Este*. London, Cambridge University Press.

Fischman HR (1982). Multiple sclerosis: a new perspective on epidemiologic patterns. *Neurology*, 32:864–870.

Flodin U et al. (1988). Multiple sclerosis, solvents and pets. A case-referent study. *Archives of Neurology*, 45:620–623.

Fog M, Hyllested K (1966). Prevalence of disseminated sclerosis in the Faroes, the Orkneys and Shetland. *Acta Neurologica Scandinavica*, 42(Suppl. 19):9–11.

Forbes RB, Swingler RJ (1999). Estimating the prevalence of multiple sclerosis in the United Kingdom by using capture–recapture methodology. *American Journal of Epidemiology*, 149, 1016–1024.

Forbes RB, Wilson SV, Swingler RJ (1999). The prevalence of multiple sclerosis in Tayside, Scotland: do latitudinal gradients really exist? *Journal of Neurology*, 246:1033–1040.

Ford HL et al. (1998). The prevalence of multiple sclerosis in the Leeds Health Authority. *Journal of Neurology, Neurosurgery and Psychiatry*, 64:605–610.

Franklin GM et al. (1988). Stress and its relationship to acute exacerbations in multiple sclerosis. *Journal of Neurologic Rehabilitation*, 2:7–11.

Fraser KB (1975). Multiple sclerosis research. In: Davidson AV, Humphrey HH, Liversedge LA, eds. *Proceedings of a joint conference of the Medical Research Council and the Multiple Sclerosis Society of Great Britain and Northern Ireland*. London, Her Majesty's Stationery Office:53–79.

French Research Group on Multiple Sclerosis (1992). Multiple sclerosis in 54 twinships: concordance rate is independent of zygosity. *Annals of Neurology*, 32:724–727.

Frerichs FT (1849). Über hirnsklerose. [Multiple sclerosis.] *Archiv für die Gesammte Medizin*, 10:334–347.

Fukazawa T et al. (1999). CTLA-4 gene polymorphisms may modulate disease in Japanese multiple sclerosis patients. *Journal of Neurological Sciences*, 171:49–55.

Gallou M et al. (1983). Epidemiologie de la sclérose en plaques en Bretagne. [Epidemiology of multiple sclerosis in Brittany.] *Presse medicine*, 12:995–999.

Garcia J et al. (1989). Prevalence of multiple sclerosis in Lanzarote (Canary Islands). *Neurology*, 39:265–267.

Gaudet JPC et al. (1995). A study of birth order and multiple sclerosis in multiplex families. *Neuroepidemiology*, 14:188–192.

Gay D, Dick G, Upton G (1986). Multiple sclerosis associated with sinusitis: case-controlled study in general practice. *Lancet*, i:815–819.

Hammond SR, English DR, McLeod JG (2000). The age-range of risk of developing multiple sclerosis: evidence from a migrant population in Australia. *Brain*, 123:968–974.

Hammond SR et al. (1987). The epidemiology of multiple sclerosis in Queensland, Australia. *Journal of Neurological Sciences*, 80:185–204.

Hammond SR et al. (1988a). The epidemiology of multiple sclerosis in 3 Australian cities: Perth, Newcastle and Hobart. *Brain*, 111:1–25.

Hammond SR et al. (1988b). The epidemiology of multiple sclerosis in western Australia. *Australian and New Zealand Journal of Medicine*, 18:102–110.

Hammond SR et al. (2000). Multiple sclerosis in Australia: prognostic factors. *Journal of Clinical Neurosciences*, 7:16–19.

Hargreaves E (1969). Epidemiological studies in Cornwall. *Proceedings of the Royal Society of Medicine*, 54:209–216.

Harvey C et al. (1994). *The economic consequences of multiple sclerosis among PVA members.* New Brunswick, NJ, Rutgers University Bureau of Economic Research.

Haupts M et al. (1994). Epidemiological data on multiple sclerosis from an industrial area in north-west Germany. In: Firnhaber W, Lauer K, eds. *Multiple sclerosis in Europe: an epidemiological update.* Darmstadt, LTV Press:143–146.

Hawkins SA, McDonnell GV (1999). Benign multiple sclerosis? Clinical course, long term follow up, and assessment of prognostic factors. *Journal of Neurology, Neurosurgery and Psychiatry*, 67:148–152.

Helmick C et al. (1989). Multiple sclerosis in Key West, Florida. *American Journal of Epidemiology*, 130:935–949.

Heltberg A, Holm NV (1982). Concordance in twins and recurrence in sibships in multiple sclerosis. *Lancet*, i:1068.

Hernandez S et al. (1995). Predictive factors of prognosis in multiple sclerosis. *Journal of Neuroimmunology Supplement*, 1:69.

Hibberd PL (1994). Use and misuse of statistics for epidemiological studies of multiple sclerosis. *Annals of Neurology*, 36(Suppl. 2):218–230.

Hoffman RE et al. (1981). Increased incidence and prevalence of multiple sclerosis in Los Alamos County, New Mexico. *Neurology*, 31:1489–1492.

Hornabrook R (1971). The prevalence of multiple sclerosis in New Zealand. *Acta Neurologica Scandinavica*, 47:426–438.

Hou JB, Zhang Z (1992). Prevalence of multiple sclerosis: a door-to-door survey in Lan Cang La Hu Zu Autonomous County, Yunnan Province of China, *Neuroepidemiology,* 11:52.

Hours M et al. (1995). The influence of pregnancy on multiple sclerosis: a European multicentric prospective study—first results. *Journal of Neuroimmunology,* September (Suppl. 1):8.

Hughes RAC et al. (1980). Pet ownership, distemper antibodies and multiple sclerosis. *Journal of Neurological Sciences,* 47:429–432.

Hung, T-P (1982). Multiple sclerosis in Taiwan: a re-appraisal. In: Kuroiwa Y, Kurland L, eds. *Multiple sclerosis: east and west,* Kyushu, Kyushu University Press:83–96.

Hutter C (1993). On the causes of multiple sclerosis. *Medical Hypotheses,* 41:93–96.

Hyllested K (1956). *Disseminated sclerosis in Denmark: prevalence and geographical distribution.* Copenhagen, J. Jorgensen & Co.

Inman RP (1984). Disability indices, the economic costs of illness, and social insurance: the case of multiple sclerosis. *Acta Neurologica Scandinavica,* 70:46–55.

Irvine DG, Schieter HB, Hader WJ (1989). Geotoxicology of multiple sclerosis: the Henribourg, Saskatchewan, Cluster Focus. I. The water. *Science of the Total Environment,* 84:45–59.

Italian Multicentre Collaborative Group (1994). The clinical course and prognosis of patients with multiple sclerosis. In: *Multiple sclerosis epidemiology: analytical approaches to the study of etiology. Abstracts from the Oslo International Think-tank on Multiple Sclerosis Epidemiology, Centre for Advanced Studies, Oslo, September 17–18, 1994.* Copenhagen, Munksgaard:40.

Izquierdo G et al. (1986). Early onset multiple sclerosis. Clinical study of 12 pathologically proven cases. *Acta Neurologica Scandinavica,* 73:493–497.

Jacobs TJ, Charles E (1980). Life events and the occurrence of cancer in children. *Psychosomatic Medicine,* 42:11–24.

Jedlicka P (1989). Epidemiology of multiple sclerosis in Czechoslovakia. In: Battaglia M, Crimi G, eds. *An update on multiple sclerosis.* Bologna, Monduzzi Editore:253–255.

Jedlicka P et al. (1994). Epidemiology of MS in the Czech Republic. In: Firnhaber W, Lauer K, eds. *Multiple sclerosis in Europe: an epidemiological update.* Darmstadt, LTV Press:261–265.

Joensen JP (1982). *Fi kafølk. [Fishermen.]* Tórshavn, Føroya Sparikassi.

Jotkowitz S (1977). Multiple sclerosis and exposure to house pets. *Journal of the American Medical Association,* 238:854.

Kahana E, Zilber N (1996). Pitfalls in multiple sclerosis epidemiology: the Israeli experience. *Neuroepidemiology*, September (Suppl. 1):9.

Kalafatova OI (1987). Geographic and climatic factors and multiple sclerosis in some districts of Bulgaria. *Neuroepidemiology*, 6:116–119.

Kantarci O et al. (1998). Survivals and predictors of disability in Turkish MS patients. Turkish Multiple Sclerosis Study Group. *Neurology*, 51:765–772.

Kaplan AS, ed. (1975). *The herpes viruses.* New York, Academic Press.

Kesselring J, Beer S (1994). Epidemiology of multiple sclerosis in Switzerland. In: Firnhaber W, Lauer K, eds. *Multiple sclerosis in Europe: an epidemiological update.* Darmstadt, LTV Press:166–167.

Khan MA, Kushner I (1979). Ankylosing spondylitis and multiple sclerosis: a possible association. *Arthritis and Rheumatism*, 22:784–786.

Kies BM (1989). An epidemiological study of multiple sclerosis in Cape Town, South Africa. In: Chopra JS, Jagannathan K, Sawhney IMS, eds. *Advances in neurology. Proceedings of the XIVth World Congress of Neurology, New Delhi, India.* Amsterdam, Excerpta Medica:278 (abstract 612B05).

Kim SW, Kim SY (1982). Multiple sclerosis in Busan, Korea. Clinical features and prevalence. In: Kuroiwa Y, Kurland LT, eds. *Multiple sclerosis: east and west,* Kyushu, Kyushu University Press:57–69.

Kinnunen E (1984). Multiple sclerosis in Finland: evidence of increasing frequency and uneven geographic distribution. *Neurology*, 34:457–461.

Kinnunen E et al. (1983). The epidemiology of multiple sclerosis in Finland: increase of prevalence and stability of foci of high risk areas. *Acta Neurologica Scandinavica*, 67:255–262.

Kinnunen E et al. (1988). Genetic susceptibility to multiple sclerosis: a co-twin study of a nation-wide series. *Archives of Neurology*, 45:1108–1111.

Klein G, Rose MS, Seland TP (1994). The prevalence of multiple sclerosis in the Crowsnest Pass region of southern Alberta. *Canadian Journal of Neurological Sciences*, 21:262–265.

Knox EG (1964). Epidemiology of childhood leukemia in Northumberland and Durham. *British Journal of Preventive and Social Medicine*, 18:17–24.

Knox EG (1977). Foods and diseases. *British Journal of Preventive and Social Medicine*, 31:71–80.

Koch MJ et al. (1974). Multiple sclerosis. A cluster in a small Northwestern United States community. *Journal of the American Medical Association*, 288:1555–1557.

Koch-Henriksen N (1995). Multiple sclerosis in Scandinavia and Finland. *Acta Neurologica Scandinavica Supplementum*, 161:55–59.

Koch-Henriksen N (1999). The Danish Multiple Sclerosis Registry: a 50-year follow-up. *Multiple Sclerosis*, 5:293–296.

Koch-Henriksen N, Hyllested K (1988). Epidemiology of multiple sclerosis: incidence and prevalence rates in Denmark 1948–64 based on the Danish Multiple Sclerosis Registry. *Acta Neurologica Scandinavica*, 78:369–380.

Koch-Henriksen N, Bronnum-Hansen K, Hyllested K (1992). Incidence of multiple sclerosis in Denmark 1948–1982: a descriptive nationwide study. *Neuroepidemiology*, 11:1–10.

Koch-Henriksen N et al. (1994). The Danish Multiple Sclerosis Registry: a 44-year review. In: Firnhaber W, Lauer K, eds. *Multiple sclerosis in Europe: an epidemiological update*. Darmstadt, LTV Press:79–86.

Koncan-Vracko B (1994). Epidemiological investigations of multiple sclerosis in Slovenia. In: Firnhaber W, Lauer K, eds. *Multiple sclerosis in Europe: an epidemiological update*. Darmstadt, LTV Press:294.

Korn-Lubetzki I et al. (1984). Activity of multiple sclerosis during pregnancy and puerperium. *Annals of Neurology*, 16:229–231.

Kraft GH et al. (1981). Multiple sclerosis: early prognostic guidelines. *Archives of Physical Medicine and Rehabilitation*, 62:54–58.

Kramer M (1957). Discussion of the context of prevalence and incidence as related to epidemiologic studies of mental disorders. *American Journal of Public Health*, 48:826.

Kranz JMS (1982). *A multiple sclerosis case-control study in Olmsted and Mower Counties, Minnesota* [Thesis]. Minneapolis MN, Graduate School of the University of Minnesota.

Kranz JMS et al. (1983). Multiple sclerosis in Olmsted and Mower Counties, Minnesota. *Neuroepidemiology*, 2:206–218.

Kreienbrock L et al. (1993). Radon and lung cancer in the Ardennes and Eifel region—concepts and experiences of an international epidemiological study. *Medical information and biometrics epidemiology* (Munich), 76:19–23.

Kruja J (1994). Multiple sclerosis in Albania: In: Firnhaber W, Lauer K, eds. *Multiple sclerosis in Europe: an epidemiological update*. Darmstadt, LTV Press:309–315.

Kruja J (1994). The natural course of multiple sclerosis in Albanian material. In: *Multiple sclerosis epidemiology: analytical approaches to the study of etiology. Abstracts from the Oslo International Think-tank on Multiple Sclerosis Epidemiology, Centre for Advanced Studies, Oslo, September 17–18, 1994*. Copenhagen, Munksgaard:38.

Kurland LT, Westlund KB (1954). Epidemiologic factors in the etiology and prognosis of multiple sclerosis. *Annals of the New York Academy of Sciences*, 58:682–701.

Kuroiwa Y et al. (1982). Clinical picture of MS in Asia. In: Kuroiwa Y, Kurland L, eds. *Multiple sclerosis: east and west*. Kyushu, Kyushu University Press:31–42.

Kuroiwa Y, Shibasaki H, Ikeda M (1983). Prevalence of MS and north-south gradient in Japan. *Neuroepidemiology*, 2:62–69.

Kurtzke JF (1965). Further notes on disability evaluation in multiple sclerosis with scale modifications. *Neurology*, 15:654–661.

Kurtzke JF (1968). A Fennoscandian focus of multiple sclerosis. *Neurology*, 18:16–20.

Kurtzke JF (1972). Migration and latency in multiple sclerosis. In: Field EJ et al., eds. *Multiple sclerosis: progress in research*. Amsterdam, North Holland.

Kurtzke JF (1974). Further features of the Fennoscandian focus of multiple sclerosis. *Acta Neurologica Scandinavica*, 50:478–502.

Kurtzke JF (1980). Epidemiologic contributions to multiple sclerosis: an overview. *Neurology*, 30:61–79.

Kurtzke JF (1985). Epidemiology of multiple sclerosis. In: Vinken PJ, Bruyn GW, Klawans HL, eds. *Handbook of clinical neurology. Vol. 47, Demyelinating diseases*. Amsterdam, Elsevier:259–287.

Kurtzke JF (1991). Multiple sclerosis: changing times. *Neuroepidemiology*, 10:1–8.

Kurtzke JF (1993). Epidemiologic evidence for multiple sclerosis as an infection. *Clinical Microbiology Reviews*, 6:382–427.

Kurtzke JF (1995). MS epidemiology world wide. One view of current status. *Acta Neurologica Scandinavica Supplementum*, 161:23–33.

Kurtzke JF (1997). The epidemiology of multiple sclerosis. In: Raine CS, McFarland HF, Tourtelotte WW, eds. *Multiple sclerosis: clinical and pathological basis*. London, Chapman & Hall Medical:91–135.

Kurtzke J, Bui QH (1980). Multiple sclerosis in a migrant population. II. Half-orientals immigrating in childhood. *Annals of Neurology*, 8:256–260.

Kurtzke JF, Hyllested K (1979). Multiple sclerosis in the Faroe Islands. I. Clinical and epidemiological features. *Annals of Neurology*, 5:6–21.

Kurtzke JF, Hyllested K (1986). Multiple sclerosis in the Faroe Islands. II. Clinical update, transmission, and the nature of MS. *Neurology*, 36:307–328.

Kurtzke JF, Hyllested K (1987). Multiple sclerosis in the Faroe Islands. III. An alternative assessment of the three epidemics. *Acta Neurologica Scandinavica*, 76:317–339.

Kurtzke JF, Beebe GW, Norman JE Jr (1979). Epidemiology of multiple sclerosis in US veterans. I. Race, sex, and geographic distribution. *Neurology*, 29:1228–1235.

Kurtzke JF, Beebe GW, Norman JE Jr (1985). Epidemiology of multiple sclerosis in US veterans. III. Migration and the risk of MS. *Neurology*, 35:672–678.

Kurtzke JF, Dean G, Botha DP (1970). A method of estimating age at immigration of white immigrants to South Africa, with an example of its importance. *South African Medical Journal*, 44:663–669.

Kurtzke JF, Delasnerie-Laupretre N, Wallin MT (1998). Multiple sclerosis in North African migrants to France. *Acta Neurologica Scandinavica*, 98:302–309.

Kurtzke JF, Guthmundsson KR, Bergmann S (1982). Multiple sclerosis in Iceland. I. Evidence of a postwar epidemic. *Neurology*, 32:143–150.

Landtblom AM et al. (1993). Multiple sclerosis and exposure to solvents, ionizing radiation, and animals. *Scandinavian Journal of Work Environment and Health*, 19:399–404.

Langmuir AD (1965). Formal discussion of epidemiology of cancer: spatial temporal aggregation. *Cancer Research*, 25:1384–1386.

LaRocca N et al. (1982). The role of disease and demographic factors in the employment of patients with multiple sclerosis. *Archives of Neurology*, 39:256.

Larsen JP et al. (1984a). Western Norway, a high-risk area for multiple sclerosis: a prevalence/incidence study in the county of Hordaland. *Neurology*, 34:1202–1207.

Larsen JP et al. (1984b). An increase in the incidence of multiple sclerosis in Western Norway. *Acta Neurologica Scandinavica*, 70:96–103.

Larsen JP et al. (1985). Clustering of multiple sclerosis in the county of Hordaland, western Norway. *Acta Neurologica Scandinavica*, 71:390–395.

Larsen JP et al. (1986). Multiple sclerosis—more than one disease. *Acta Neurologica Scandinavica*, 72:145–150.

Lauer K (1989). Multiple sclerosis in relation to meat preservation in France and Switzerland. *Neuroepidemiology*, 8:308–315.

Lauer K (1991). The food pattern in geographical relation to the risk of multiple sclerosis in the Mediterranean and Near East region. *Journal of Epidemiology and Community Health*, 45:251–252.

Lauer K (1994). The risk of multiple sclerosis in the U.S.A. in relation to sociogeographic features: a factor-analytic study. *Journal of Clinical Epidemiology*, 47:43–48.

Lauer K (1995). Environmental associations with the risk of multiple sclerosis: the contribution of ecological studies. *Acta Neurologica Scandinavica Supplementum*, 161:77–88.

Lauer K, Firnhaber W (1992). Die multiple-sklerose-mortalität 1973–1987 in Baden-Württemberg im Vergleich mit soziogeographischen Variablen. [Multiple sclerosis mortality 1973–1987 in Baden-Württemberg in comparison with socio-geographical variables.] *Nervenarzt*, 63:209–212.

Lauer K, Firnhaber W (1994). Descriptive and analytical epidemiological data on multiple sclerosis from a long-term study in Southern Hesse, Germany. In: Firnhaber W, Lauer K, eds. *Multiple sclerosis in Europe: an epidemiological update*. Darmstadt, LTV Press:147–158.

Leibowitz U, Alter M (1973). *Multiple sclerosis: clues to its cause*. Amsterdam, North Holland.

Leibowitz U, Kahana E, Alter M (1969). Multiple sclerosis in immigrant and native populations of Israel. *Lancet*, i:1323–1325.

Leibowitz U et al. (1972). The cause of death in multiple sclerosis. In: Leibowitz U, ed. *Progress in multiple sclerosis*. New York, Academic Press:196–209.

Levic ZM et al. (1999). Prognostic factors for survival in multiple sclerosis. *Multiple Sclerosis*, 5:171–178.

Lilienfeld DE, Stolley PD (1994). *Foundations of epidemiology*, 3rd ed. New York, Oxford University Press.

Limburg CC (1950). The geographic distribution of multiple sclerosis and its estimated prevalence in the United States. *Proceedings of the Association for Research on Nervous and Mental Diseases*, 28:15–24.

Logsdail SJ, Callanan MM, Ron MA (1988). Psychiatric morbidity in patients with clinically isolated lesions of the type seen in multiple sclerosis: a clinical and MRI study. *Psychological Medicine*, 18:355–364.

Lyon-Caen O et al. (1985). Late onset multiple sclerosis: clinical study of 16 pathologically proven cases. *Acta Neurologica Scandinavica*, 72:56–60.

Mackay RP, Myrianthopoulos NC (1966). Multiple sclerosis in twins and their relatives. *Archives of Neurology and Psychiatry*, 15:449–462.

Malosse D, Perron H (1993). Correlation analysis between bovine populations, other farm animals, house pets, and multiple sclerosis prevalence. *Neuroepidemiology*, 12:15–27.

Mantel N (1967). The detection of disease clustering and a generalized regression approach. *Cancer Research*, 27:209–220.

Margolis LN, Graves RW (1945). The occurrence of myasthenia gravis in a patient with multiple sclerosis. *North Carolina Medical Journal*, 6:243–244.

Massey EW, Schoenberg BS (1982). International patterns of mortality from multiple sclerosis. *Neuroepidemiology*, 1:189–196.

Materljan E et al. (1989). Multiple sclerosis in Istria, Yugoslavia. *Neurologija*, 38:201–212.

Matias-Guiu J et al. (1994). A matched case-control study on multiple sclerosis in Alcoi, Spain. In: Firnhaber W, Lauder K, eds. *Multiple sclerosis in Europe: an epidemiological update*. Darmstadt, LTV Press:190–191.

Matthews WB (1985). Clinical aspects of multiple sclerosis: course and prognosis. In: Matthews WB et al., eds. *McAlpine's multiple sclerosis*. Edinburgh, Churchill Livingstone, Chapter 3.

McAlpine D (1961). The benign form of multiple sclerosis: a study based on 241 cases seen within three years of onset and followed up until the tenth year or more of the disease. *Brain*, 84:186–203.

McAlpine D (1972). The problem of diagnosis. In: McAlpine D, Lumsden C, Acheson ED, eds. *Multiple sclerosis: a reappraisal*. Edinburgh, Churchill Livingstone:224–257.

McAlpine D (1985). Laboratory diagnosis. In: Matthews WB et al., eds. *McAlpine's multiple sclerosis*. Edinburgh, Churchill Livingstone, Chapter 8.

McAlpine D, Compston ND (1952). Some aspects of the natural history of disseminated sclerosis. *Quarterly Journal of Medicine*, 21:135–167.

McAlpine D et al. (1955). *Multiple sclerosis*. Edinburgh, Livingstone.

McCall MG et al. (1968). Frequency of multiple sclerosis in three Australian cities—Perth, Newcastle and Hobart. *Journal of Neurology, Neurosurgery and Psychiatry*, 31:1–9.

McDonald WI, Halliday AM (1977). Diagnosis and classification of multiple sclerosis. *British Medical Bulletin*, 33:4–9.

McDonnell GV, Hawkins SA (1998). An epidemiologic study of multiple sclerosis in Northern Ireland. *Neurology*, 50:423–428.

McDonnell GV et al. (1999). A study of the HLA-DR region in clinical subgroups of multiple sclerosis and its influence on prognosis. *Journal of Neurological Sciences*, 165:77–83.

McLeod JG, Hammond SR, Hallpike JF (1994). Epidemiology of multiple sclerosis in Australia. With NSW and SA survey results. *Medical Journal of Australia*, 160:117–122.

Medaer R (1979). Does the history of multiple sclerosis go back as far as the 14th century? *Acta Neurologica Scandinavica*, 60:189–192.

Meneghini F et al. (1991). Door-to-door prevalence survey of neurological diseases in a Sicilian population. Background and methods. The Sicilian Neuro-Epidemiologic Study Group. *Neuroepidemiology*, 10:70–85.

Meucci G et al. (1992). Indagine sulla prevalenza della sclerosi multipla nel USL n. 17 del Valdarno inferiore. [Investigation into the prevalence of multiple sclerosis in local health centre no. 17 of Lower Valdarno.] In: *VII Convegno Nazionale di Neuroepidemiologia, abstract book*. Perugia, Tipografia Umbria:35.

Meyer-Rienecker H (1994). Epidemiological analyses on multiple sclerosis in the region of Rostock, north-east Germany. In: Firnhaber W, Lauer K, eds. *Multiple sclerosis in Europe: an epidemiological update*. Darmstadt, LTV Press:143–146.

Meyer-Rienecker H, Buddenhagen F (1988). Incidence of multiple sclerosis: a periodic or stable phenomenon. *Journal of Neurology*, 235:241–244.

Middleton LT, Dean G (1991). Multiple sclerosis in Cyprus. *Journal of Neurological Sciences*, 103:29–36.

Midgard R, Riise T, Nyland H (1991). Epidemiologic trends in multiple sclerosis in Møre and Romsdal, Norway: a prevalence/incidence study in a stable population. *Neurology*, 41:887–892.

Midgard R, Riise T, Nyland H (1994). Incidence of multiple sclerosis: a population-based, longitudinal study in Møre and Romsdal, Norway. In: Firnhaber W, Lauer K, eds. *Multiple sclerosis in Europe: an epidemiological update*. Darmstadt, LTV Press:67–69.

Milanov I et al. (1997). Prevalence of multiple sclerosis in Bulgaria. *Neuroepidemiology*, 16:304–307.

Milanov I et al. (1999). Prevalence of multiple sclerosis in Gypsies and Bulgarians. *Neuroepidemiology*, 18:218–222.

Millar JHD (1966). Multiple sclerosis, two high risk areas in Northern Ireland. *Journal of the Irish Medical Association*, 59:138–143.

Millar JHD (1972). *Multiple sclerosis: a disease acquired in childhood?* Springfield, Charles C. Thomas.

Millar JHD, Allison RS (1954). Familial incidence of disseminated sclerosis in Northern Ireland. *Ulster Medical Journal*, 23(Suppl. 2):29–92.

Millar JHD et al. (1959). Pregnancy as a factor influencing relapse in disseminated sclerosis. *Brain*, 82:417–426.

Miller DH et al. (1990). Multiple sclerosis in Australia and New Zealand: are the determinants genetic or environmental? *Journal of Neurology, Neurosurgery and Psychiatry*, 53:903–905.

Miller H et al. (1960). Multiple sclerosis: a note on social incidence. *British Medical Journal*, 2:343–345.

Milonas I, Tsounis S, Logothetis I (1990). Epidemiology of multiple sclerosis in northern Greece. *Acta Neurologica Scandinavica*, 81:43–47.

Minderhoud J, Zwanniken C (1994). Increasing prevalence and incidence of multiple sclerosis: an epidemiological study in the province of Groningen, The Netherlands. In: Firnhaber W, Lauer K, eds. *Multiple sclerosis in Europe: an epidemiological update*. Darmstadt, LTV Press:113–121.

Minuk GY, Lewkonia RM (1986). Possible familial association of multiple sclerosis and inflammatory bowel disease. *New England Journal of Medicine*, 314:586.

Moreau T et al. (1995). PRESTIMUS: predictive estimates in multiple sclerosis. A European multicentric prospective study. *Journal of Neuroimmunology*, September (Suppl. 1):8.

Moreau T et al. (2000). Incidence of multiple sclerosis in Dijon, France: a population-based ascertainment. *Neurological research*, 22:156–159.

Moresco M, Rossi G (1989). Studie di prevalenza della sclerosi multipla nella USL Vallagarina-Rovereto. [Study of the prevalence of multiple sclerosis in Vallagarina-Rovereto.] In: Battaglia MA, Crimi G, eds. *An update on multiple sclerosis*. Bologna, Monduzzi Editore:287–291.

Morganti G et al. (1984). Multiple sclerosis in the Republic of San Marino. *Journal of Epidemiology and Community Health*, 38:23–28.

Moxon D (1875). Eight cases of insular sclerosis of the brain and spinal cord. *Guy's Hospital Report*, 20:437–478.

Muller R (1949). Studies on disseminated sclerosis, with special reference to symptomatology, course and prognosis. *Acta Medica Scandinavica*, 133(Suppl. 222):1–214.

Muller R (1953). Genetic aspects of multiple sclerosis. *Archives of Neurology and Psychiatry, Chicago*, 70:733–740.

Mumford CJ et al. (1992). Multiple sclerosis in the Cambridge health district of East Anglia. *Journal of Neurology, Neurosurgery and Psychiatry*, 55:877–882.

Mumford CJ et al. (1994). The British Isles survey of multiple sclerosis in twins. *Neurology*, 44:11–15.

Murray TJ (1976). An unusual occurrence of multiple sclerosis in a small rural community. *Canadian Journal of Neurological Sciences*, 3:163–166.

Murrell TGC, Matthews BJ (1990). Multiple sclerosis—one manifestation of neurobrucellosis? *Medical Hypotheses*, 33:43–44.

Mutlu T (1960). The effect of geographical and meteorological factors on the incidence of multiple sclerosis in Turkey. *Acta Neurologica Scandinavica*, 35(Suppl. 147):47–54.

Myhr KM et al. (1994). Long-term prognosis in an incidence cohort of 219 multiple sclerosis patients from Hordaland County, western Norway. In: *Multiple sclerosis epidemiology: analytical approaches to the study of etiology. Abstracts from the Oslo International Think-tank on Multiple Sclerosis Epidemiology, Centre for Advanced Studies, Oslo, September 17–18, 1994.* Copenhagen, Munksgaard:39.

Namerow NS, Thompson LR (1969). Plaques, symptoms and the remitting course of multiple sclerosis. *Neurology*, 19:765–774.

Nanji AA, Narod S (1986). Multiple sclerosis, latitude and dietary fat: is pork the missing link? *Medical Hypotheses*, 20:279–282.

Nardozza V et al. (1988). Prevalence of multiple sclerosis in the town of Biella, northern Italy. In: *1988 International Multiple Sclerosis Conference, abstract book.* Rome, Italian Multiple Sclerosis Association:IV/37.

Nathanson N (1980). Slow viruses and chronic disease: the contribution of epidemiology. *Public Health Report*, 95:436–443.

Nelson LM, Franklin GM, Jones MC (1988). Risk of multiple sclerosis exacerbation during pregnancy and breast-feeding. *Journal of the American Medical Association*, 259:3441–3443.

Norman JE Jr, Cook SD, Dowling PC (1983). Pilot survey of household pets among veterans with multiple sclerosis and age-matched controls. Pilot survey. *Archives of Neurology*, 40:213–214.

Noseworthy J et al. (1983). Multiple sclerosis after 50. *Neurology*, 33:1537–1544.

Oftedal S (1966). Multiple sclerosis in Vestfold, Norway. *Acta Neurologica Scandinavica*, 42(Suppl. 19):19–25.

Page WF et al. (1993). Epidemiology of multiple sclerosis in U.S. veterans. V. Ancestry and the risk of MS. *Annals of Neurology*, 33:632–639.

Page WF et al. (1995). Epidemiology of multiple sclerosis in US veterans. VI. Population ancestry and surname ethnicity as risk factors for multiple sclerosis. *Neuroepidemiology*, 14:286–296.

Palffy G (1982). MS in Hungary, including the Gypsy population. In: Kuroiwa Y, Kurland L, eds. *Multiple sclerosis: east and west.* Kyushu, Kyushu University Press:149–157.

Palffy G (1988). The validity of diagnostic criteria in multiple sclerosis. *Acta Medica Hungary*, 45:63–71.

Palffy G et al. (1994). Multiple sclerosis in Baranya County in Hungarians and in Gypsies. In: Firnhaber W, Lauer K, eds. *Multiple sclerosis in Europe: an epidemiological update.* Darmstadt, LTV Press:274–278.

Palo J, Wikström J, Kivalo E (1973). Further studies on the epidemiology of multiple sclerosis in Finland. *Acta Neurologica Scandinavica,* 49:495–501.

Panelius M (1969). Studies on epidemiological, clinical and etiological aspects of multiple sclerosis. *Acta Neurologica Scandinavica,* 45(Suppl. 39):1–82.

Park C (1966). Multiple sclerosis in Korea. *Neurology,* 16:919–926.

Percy AK et al. (1971). Multiple sclerosis in Rochester, Minnesota. A 60-year appraisal. *Archives of Neurology,* 25:105–111.

Petrescu A (1994). Epidemiology of multiple sclerosis in Romania. In: Firnhaber W, Lauer K, eds. *Multiple sclerosis in Europe: an epidemiological update.* Darmstadt, LTV Press:287–293.

Phadke JG, Downie AW (1987). Epidemiology of multiple sclerosis in the north-east (Grampian region) of Scotland—an update. *Journal of Epidemiology and Community Health,* 41:5–13.

Piazza A et al. (1988). A genetic history of Italy. *Annals of Human Genetics,* 52:203–213.

Pina MA et al. (1998). Prevalence of multiple sclerosis in the sanitary district of Calatayud, Northern Spain: is Spain a zone of high risk for this disease? *Neuroepidemiology,* 17:258–264.

Poser CM (1987). Trauma and multiple sclerosis. An hypothesis. *Journal of Neurology,* 254:155–159.

Poser CM (1994). The epidemiology of multiple sclerosis: a general overview. *Annals of Neurology,* 36(Suppl. 2):S180–S193.

Poser CM (1995). Viking voyages: the origin of multiple sclerosis? An essay in medical history. *Acta Neurologica Scandinavica Supplementum,* 91:11–22.

Poser CM, Benedikz J, Hibberd PL (1992). The epidemiology of multiple sclerosis: the Iceland model. *Journal of Neurological Sciences,* 111:143–152.

Poser CM et al. (1983). New diagnostic criteria for multiple sclerosis. *Annals of Neurology,* 13:227–231.

Poser S (1994). The epidemiology of multiple sclerosis in southern Lower Saxony. In: Firnhaber W, Lauer K, eds. *Multiple sclerosis in Europe: an epidemiological update.* Darmstadt, LTV Press:130–133.

Poser S, Poser W (1983). Multiple sclerosis and gestation. *Neurology,* 331:1422–1427.

Poser S, Raun NE, Poser W (1982). Age at onset, initial symptomatology and the course of multiple sclerosis. *Acta Neurologica Scandinavica*, 66:355–362.

Poser S et al. (1979). Pregnancy, oral contraceptives and multiple sclerosis. *Acta Neurologica Scandinavica*, 59:108–118.

Poskanzer DC (1965). Tonsillectomy in multiple sclerosis. *Lancet*, ii:1264–1266.

Poskanzer DC, Prenney LB, Sheridan JL (1977). House pets and multiple sclerosis. *Lancet*, i:1204.

Poskanzer DC, Schapira K, Miller H (1963a). Epidemiology of multiple sclerosis in the counties of Northumberland and Durham. *Journal of Neurology, Neurosurgery and Psychiatry*, 26:368–376.

Poskanzer DC, Schapira K, Miller H (1963b). Multiple sclerosis and poliomyelitis. *Lancet*, ii:917–921.

Poskanzer DC et al. (1980a). Multiple sclerosis in the Orkney and Shetland Islands. I. Epidemiology, clinical factors, and methodology. *Journal of Epidemiology and Community Health*, 34:229–239.

Poskanzer DC et al. (1980b). Multiple sclerosis in the Orkney and Shetland Islands. II. The search for an exogenous aetiology. *Journal of Epidemiology and Community Health*, 34:240–252.

Poskanzer DC et al. (1981). The etiology of multiple sclerosis: temporal-spatial clustering indicating two environmental exposures before onset. *Neurology*, 6:708–713.

Potemkowski A et al. (1994). Epidemiological analysis of multiple sclerosis in the Szczecin region, north-western part of Poland (1962–1992). In: Firnhaber W, Lauer K, eds. *Multiple sclerosis in Europe: an epidemiological update*. Darmstadt, LTV Press:249–254.

Prange AGA et al. (1986). Epidemiological aspects of multiple sclerosis: a comparative study of four centres in Europe. *Neuroepidemiology*, 5:71–79.

Pratt RTC (1951). An investigation of the psychiatric aspects of disseminated sclerosis. *Journal of Neurology, Neurosurgery and Psychiatry*, 14:326–335.

Pryse-Phillips WE (1986). The incidence and prevalence of multiple sclerosis in Newfoundland and Labrador, 1960–1984. *Annals of Neurology*, 20:323–328.

Rabins PV et al. (1986). Structural brain correlates of emotional disorder in multiple sclerosis. *Brain*, 109:585–597.

Radhakrishnan K et al. (1985). Prevalence and pattern of multiple sclerosis in Benghazi, north-eastern Libya. *Journal of Neurological Sciences*, 70:39–46.

Rang EH, Brooke BN, Hermon-Taylor J (1982). Association of ulcerative colitis with multiple sclerosis. *Lancet*, ii:555.

Read D et al. (1982). Multiple sclerosis and dog ownership. A case-control investigation. *Journal of Neurological Sciences*, 55:359–367.

Resch J (1994). Relation in space and time between the frequency of multiple sclerosis and geophysical factors. In: Firnhaber W, Lauer K, eds. *Multiple sclerosis in Europe: an epidemiological update*. Darmstadt, LTV Press:159–165.

Rewers M et al. (1988). Trends in the prevalence and incidence of diabetes: insulin-dependent diabetes mellitus in childhood. *World Health Statistics Quarterly*, 41:179–189.

Rice-Oxley M, William ES, Rees JE (1995). A prevalence survey of multiple sclerosis in Sussex. *Journal of Neurology, Neurosurgery and Psychiatry*, 58:27–30.

Riise T et al. (1991). Clustering of residence of multiple sclerosis patients at age 13 to 20 years in Hordaland, Norway. *American Journal of Epidemiology*, 133:932–939.

Roberson PK (1990). Controlling for time-varying population distributions in disease clustering studies. *American Journal of Epidemiology*, 132(Suppl. 1):S131–S135.

Roberts DF (1986). Multiple sclerosis in the Orkney and Shetlands Islands. In: Rose C, ed. *Clinical neuroepidemiology*. Baltimore, MD, University Park Press.

Roberts DF, Bates D (1982). The genetic contribution to multiple sclerosis—evidence from north-east England. *Journal of Neurological Sciences*, 54:287–293.

Roberts DF, Roberts MJ, Poskanzer DC (1979). Genetic analysis of multiple sclerosis in Orkney. *Journal of Epidemiology and Community Health*, 33:229–235.

Roberts MHW et al. (1991). The prevalence of multiple sclerosis in the Southampton and South West Hampshire Health Authority. *Journal of Neurology, Neurosurgery and Psychiatry*, 53:55–59.

Robertson N, Compston D (1995). Surveying multiple sclerosis in the United Kingdom. *Journal of Neurology, Neurosurgery and Psychiatry*, 58:2–6.

Rogers MP, Dubey D, Reich P (1979). The influence of the psyche and the brain on immunity and disease susceptibility: a critical review. *Psychosomatic Medicine*, 41:147–164.

Rosati G (1994). Descriptive epidemiology of multiple sclerosis in Europe in the 1980s. A critical review. *Annals of Neurology*, 36(Suppl. 2):S164–S174.

Rosati G et al. (1986). Incidence of multiple sclerosis in Macomer, Sardinia, 1912–1981: onset of the disease after 1950. *Neurology*, 36:14–19.

Rosati G et al. (1987). Sardinia, a high-risk area for multiple sclerosis: a prevalence and incidence study in the district of Alghero. *Annals of Neurology*, 21:190–194.

Rosati G et al. (1988). Incidence of multiple sclerosis in the town of Sassari, Sardinia, 1965 to 1985: evidence for increasing occurrence of the disease. *Neurology*, 38:384–388.

Rosati G et al. (1991). Prevalence and incidence study of multiple sclerosis in the district of Tempio, Sardinia, 1960 to 1986. *Italian Journal of Neurological Sciences*, 12(Suppl. 5):28.

Rosati G et al. (1996). Epidemiology of multiple sclerosis in Northwestern Sardinia: further evidence for higher frequency in Sardinians compared to other Italians. *Neuroepidemiology*, 15:10–19.

Rose AS et al. (1976). Criteria for the clinical diagnosis of multiple sclerosis. *Neurology*, 26:20–22.

Rosman K, Jacobs HA, van der Merwe CA (1985). A new multiple sclerosis epidemic? A pilot survey. *South African Medical Journal*, 68:162–163.

Roth MP et al. (1994). Multiple sclerosis in the Pyrenées-Atlantique: a case-control study conducted in the southwest of France. In: Firnhaber W, Lauer K, eds. *Multiple sclerosis in Europe: an epidemiological update*. Darmstadt, LTV Press:177–178.

Rothman KJ (1986). *Modern epidemiology*. Boston, MA, Little, Brown.

Rothman KJ (1990). A sobering start for the cluster busters' conference. *American Journal of Epidemiology*, 132(Suppl. 1):S6–S13.

Rothwell PM, Charlton D (1998). High incidence and prevalence of multiple sclerosis in south east Scotland: evidence of a genetic predisposition. *Journal of Neurology, Neurosurgery and Psychiatry*, 64:730–735.

Rudez J et al. (1995). Associated diseases and multiple sclerosis in Croatia. In: *Multiple sclerosis epidemiology; analytical approaches to the study of etiology. Abstracts from the Oslo International Think-tank on Multiple Sclerosis Epidemiology, Centre for Advanced Studies, Oslo, September 17–18, 1994*. Copenhagen, Munksgaard:11.

Runmarker B, Andersen O (1993). Prognostic factors in multiple sclerosis incidence cohort with twenty five years of follow-up. *Brain*, 116:117–134.

Runmarker B, Andersen O (1995). Pregnancy is associated with a lower risk of onset and a better prognosis in multiple sclerosis. *Brain*, 118:253–261.

Sadovnick AD (1994). Genetic epidemiology of multiple sclerosis: a survey. *Annals of Neurology*, 36(Suppl. 2):S194–S203.

Sadovnick AD, Ebers GC (1993). Epidemiology of multiple sclerosis: a critical overview. *Canadian Journal of Neurological Sciences*, 20:17–29.

Sadovnick AD, Baird PA, Ward RH (1988). Multiple sclerosis: updated risks for relatives. *American Journal of Medical Genetics*, 29:533–541.

Sadovnick AD et al. (1991). The influence of gender on susceptibility to multiple sclerosis in sibships. *Archives of Neurology*, 48:586–588.

Sadovnick AD et al. (1993). A population-based study of multiple sclerosis in twins: update. *Annals of Neurology*, 33:281–285.

Sadovnick AD et al. (1996). Evidence for the genetic basis of multiple sclerosis. *Lancet*, 347:1728–1730.

Savettieri G et al. (1981). The prevalence of multiple sclerosis in Sicily. I. Monreale city. *Journal of Epidemiology and Community Health*, 35:114–117.

Savettieri G et al. (1986). A further study on the prevalence of multiple sclerosis in Sicily: Caltanissetta city. *Acta Neurologica Scandinavica*, 73:71–75.

Schapira K, Poskanzer DC, Miller H (1963). Familial and conjugal multiple sclerosis. *Brain*, 86:315–332.

Schapira K et al. (1966). Marriage, pregnancy and multiple sclerosis. *Brain*, 89:419–428.

Scheinberg L et al. (1980). Multiple sclerosis: earning a living. *New York State Journal of Medicine*, August:1395–1400.

Schiffer RB et al. (1994). A genetic marker and family history study of the upstate New York multiple sclerosis cluster. *Neurology*, 44:329–333.

Schmidt R et al. (1989). Frequency and distribution of MS in the district of Halle. In: Battaglia M, Crimi G, eds. *An update on multiple sclerosis*. Bologna, Monduzzi Editore:303–305.

Schonberger LB et al. (1981). Guillain-Barré syndrome: its epidemiology and association with influenza vaccination. *Annals of Neurology*, 9(Suppl. 1):31–38.

Schottenfeld D, Fraumeni JF (1982). *Cancer epidemiology and prevention*. Philadelphia, WB Saunders.

Schumacher GA et al. (1965). Problems of experimental trials of therapy in multiple sclerosis; report by the panel on the evaluation of experimental trials of therapy in multiple sclerosis. *Annals of the New York Academy of Sciences*, 122:552–568.

Seguin EC, Shaw JC, Van Derveer A (1878). A contribution to the pathological anatomy of disseminated cerebro-spinal sclerosis. *Journal of Nervous and Mental Disease*, 5:281–293.

Sepcic J et al. (1989). Multiple sclerosis cluster in Gorski Kotar, Croatia, Yugoslavia. In: Battaglia M, ed. *Multiple sclerosis research*. Amsterdam, Elsevier:165–169.

Sepcic J et al. (1993). Nutritional factors and multiple sclerosis in Gorski Kotar, Croatia. *Neuroepidemiology*, 12:234–240.

Shakir RA, Hussein JM, Trontelj JV (1983). Myasthenia gravis and multiple sclerosis. *Journal of Neuroimmunology*, 4:161–165.

Sharpe G et al. (1995). Multiple sclerosis in island populations: prevalence in the Bailiwicks of Guernsey and Jersey. *Journal of Neurology, Neurosurgery and Psychiatry*, 58:22–26.

Shatin R (1964). Multiple sclerosis and geography. New interpretation of epidemiological observations. *Neurology*, 14:335–344.

Shepherd DI (1991). Increased risk of multiple sclerosis among doctors and nurses. *Journal of Neurology, Neurosurgery and Psychiatry*, 54:848.

Shepherd DI, Downie AW (1980). A further prevalence study of multiple sclerosis in north east Scotland. *Journal of Neurology, Neurosurgery and Psychiatry*, 43:310–315.

Shibasaki H, Okihiro MM, Kuroiwa Y (1978). Multiple sclerosis among Orientals and Caucasians in Hawaii: a reappraisal. *Neurology*, 28:113–118.

Sibley WA (1988). Risk factors in multiple sclerosis—implication for pathogenesis. In: Serlupi Crescenzi G, ed. *A multidisciplinary approach to myelin diseases.* New York, Plenum Press:227–232.

Sibley WA, Bamford CA, Clark K (1985). Clinical viral infections and multiple sclerosis. *Lancet*, ii:1313–1315.

Sibley WA et al. (1991). A prospective study of physical trauma and multiple sclerosis. *Journal of Neurology, Neurosurgery and Psychiatry*, 54:584–589.

Siedler H et al. (1958). The prevalence and incidence of multiple sclerosis in Missoula County, Montana. *Journal-Lancet (Minneapolis)*, 78:358–360.

Sironi L et al. (1991). Frequency of multiple sclerosis in Valle d'Aosta, 1971–1985. *Neuroepidemiology*, 10:66–69.

Siva A et al. (1993). Trauma and multiple sclerosis: a population-based cohort study from Olmsted County, Minnesota. *Neurology*, 43:1878–1882.

Skegg DCG et al. (1987). Occurrence of multiple sclerosis at the north and south of New Zealand. *Journal of Neurology, Neurosurgery and Psychiatry*, 50:134–139.

Stazio A, Paddison RM, Kurland LT (1967). Multiple sclerosis in New Orleans, Louisiana, and Winnipeg, Manitoba, Canada: follow-up of a previous survey in New Orleans, and comparison between the patient populations in the two communities. *Journal of Chronic Diseases*, 20:311–332.

Stazio A et al. (1964). Multiple sclerosis in Winnipeg, Manitoba: methodological consideration of epidemiologic survey: ten-year follow-up of a community-wide study and population resurvey. *Journal of Chronic Diseases*, 17:415–438.

Steiner G (1938). Multiple sclerosis. I: The etiological significance of the regional and occupational incidence. *Journal of Nervous and Mental Disease*, 88:42–66.

Steinman L (1993). Autoimmune disease. *Scientific American*, September:107–114.

Sternfeld L (1995). *Utilization and perceptions of healthcare services by people with MS*. New York, US National Multiple Sclerosis Society.

Sullivan CB, Visscher BR, Detels R (1984). Multiple sclerosis and age of exposure to childhood diseases and animals: cases and their friends. *Neurology*, 34:1144–1148.

Sumelahti ML et al. (2000). Regional and temporal variation in the incidence of multiple sclerosis in Finland 1979–1993. *Neuroepidemiology*, 19:67–75.

Sutherland JM (1956). Observations on the prevalence of multiple sclerosis in northern Scotland. *Brain*, 79:635–654.

Svenningsson A et al. (1990). Incidence of MS during two fifteen-year periods in the Gothenburg region of Sweden. *Acta Neurologica Scandinavica*, 82:161–168.

Svenson LW, Woodhead SE, Platt GH (1994). Regional variations in the prevalence rates of multiple sclerosis in the province of Alberta, Canada. *Neuroepidemiology*, 13:8–13.

Swank RL (1961). *A biochemical approach to multiple sclerosis*. Springfield, Charles C Thomas.

Swank RL et al. (1952). Multiple sclerosis in rural Norway. *New England Journal of Medicine*, 246:721–728.

Sweeney VP, Sadovnick AD, Brandejs V (1986). Prevalence of multiple sclerosis in British Columbia. *Canadian Journal of Neurological Sciences*, 13:47–51.

Sweeney WJ (1955). Pregnancy and multiple sclerosis. *American Journal of Obstetrics and Gynecology*, 66:124–130.

Swingler RJ, Compston DAS (1988). The prevalence of multiple sclerosis in south east Wales. *Journal of Neurology, Neurosurgery and Psychiatry*, 51:1520–1524.

Sylwester DL, Poser CM (1979). The association of multiple sclerosis with domestic animals and household pets. *Annals of Neurology*, 5:207–208.

Tan C (1988). Multiple sclerosis in Malaysia. *Archives of Neurology*, 45:624–627.

Thorogood M, Hannaford PC (1998). The influence of oral contraceptives on the risk of multiple sclerosis. *British Journal of Obstetrics and Gynaecology*, 105:1296–1299.

Tillman A (1950). The effect of pregnancy on multiple sclerosis and its management. *Research Publications of the Association for Research into Nervous and Mental Disease*, 28:548–582.

Torrey EF (1987). Prevalence studies in schizophrenia. *British Journal of Psychiatry*, 150:598–608.

Torrey EF, Rawlings R, Waldman IN (1988). Schizophrenic births and viral diseases in two states. *Schizophrenia Research*, 1:73–77.

Totaro R et al. (2000). Prevalence of multiple sclerosis in the L'Aquila district, central Italy. *Journal of Neurology, Neurosurgery and Psychiatry*, 68:349–352.

Trostle DC, Helfrich D, Medsger TA Jr (1986). Systemic sclerosis (scleroderma) and multiple sclerosis. *Arthritis and Rheumatism*, 29:124–127.

Ulett G (1946). Geographic distribution of multiple sclerosis. *Diseases of the Nervous System*, 9:342–346.

Uria D et al. (1994). Prevalence and incidence of multiple sclerosis in Europe: an epidemiological update. In: Firnhaber W, Lauer K, eds. *Multiple sclerosis in Europe: an epidemiological update*. Darmstadt, LTV Press:179–183.

Van Lambalgen R, Sanders EA, D'Amaro J (1986). Sex distribution, age of onset and HLA profiles in two types of multiple sclerosis. A role for sex hormones and microbial infections in the development of autoimmunity? *Journal of Neurological Sciences*, 76:13–21.

Van Ooteghem P et al. (1994). Prevalence of multiple sclerosis in Flanders, Belgium. *Neuroepidemiology*, 13:220–225.

Vassallo L, Elian M, Dean G (1979). Multiple sclerosis in southern Europe. II. Prevalence in Malta in 1978. *Journal of Epidemiology and Community Health*, 33:111–113.

Visscher BR et al. (1977). Latitude, migration, and the prevalence of multiple sclerosis. *American Journal of Epidemiology*, 106:470–475.

Von Wilhelm E (1970). Beziehungen zwischen Erkrankungen ins Kindesalter und Multiple-Sklerose-Erkrankung. [Relationship between diseases in childhood and multiple sclerosis.] *Schweizer Archiv für Neurologie, Neurchirurgie und Psychiatrie*, 106:311–317.

Wadia N, Bhatia K (1990). MS is prevalent in the Zoroastrians (Parsis) of India. *Annals of Neurology*, 28:177–179.

Warren HV, Delavault RE, Cross CH (1967). Possible correlations between geology and some disease patterns. *Annals of the New York Academy of Sciences*, 136:659–710.

Warren KG, Catz I, Steinman L (1995). Fine specificity of the antibody response to myelin basic protein in the central nervous system in multiple sclerosis: the minimal B-cell epitope and a model of its features. *Proceedings of the National Academy of Sciences of the United States of America*, 92:11061–11065.

Warren KG et al. (1994). Anti-myelin basic protein and anti-proteolipid protein specific forms of multiple sclerosis. *Annals of Neurology*, 35:280–289.

Warren S, Warren KG (1981). Multiple sclerosis and related diseases: a relationship to diabetes mellitus. *Canadian Journal of Neurological Sciences*, 8:35–39.

Warren S, Warren KG (1982). Multiple sclerosis and diabetes mellitus: further evidence of a relationship. *Canadian Journal of Neurological Sciences*, 9:415–419.

Warren S, Warren KG (1992). Prevalence of multiple sclerosis in Barrhead County, Alberta, Canada. *Canadian Journal of Neurological Sciences*, 19:72–75.

Warren S, Warren KG (1993). Prevalence, incidence, and characteristics of multiple sclerosis in Westlock County, Alberta, Canada. *Neurology*, 43:1760–1763.

Warren S, Warren KG (1995). Epidemiological features of two immunologically distinct forms of multiple sclerosis (MS): anti-myelin basic (MBP) associated MS vs anti-proteolipid (PLP) associated MS. *Journal of Neuroimmunology*, September(Suppl. 1):9.

Warren S, Warren KG (1996). Influence of gender on susceptibility to multiple sclerosis and age of onset in concordant sibships. *International Journal of Epidemiology*, 25:142–145.

Warren S, Cockerill R, Warren KG (1991). Risk factors by onset age in multiple sclerosis. *Neuroepidemiology*, 10:9–17.

Warren S, Warren KG, Cockerill R (1991). Emotional stress and coping in multiple sclerosis (MS) exacerbations. *Journal of Psychosomatic Research*, 35:37–47.

Warren S, Warren KG, Svenson L (1999). Mortality rates for multiple sclerosis (MS) in Canada, 1965–94. *Neuroepidemiology*, 18:331–332.

Warren S et al. (1982). How multiple sclerosis is related to animal illness, stress, and diabetes. *Canadian Medical Association Journal*, 126:377–385.

Warren S et al. (1984). Risk factors associated with different onset ages in multiple sclerosis patients. *Neurology*, 34(Suppl. 1):154.

Warren S et al. (1985a). Predicting the development of multiple sclerosis following an attack of optic neuritis. *Journal of Neurology*, 232:75.

Warren S et al. (1985b). Predicting the course of multiple sclerosis: factors which may be associated with disability. *Canadian Journal of Neurological Sciences*, 12:203.

Warren S et al. (1993a). Do MS risk factors vary by gender? *Neuroepidemiology*, 12:20.

Warren S et al. (1993b). Clinical features and risk factors in familial versus sporadic multiple sclerosis. *Schweizer Archiv für Neurologie und Psychiatrie*, 144:317.

Warren S et al. (1996). Parental ancestry and risk of multiple sclerosis in Alberta, Canada. *Neuroepidemiology*, 15:1–9.

Wechsler IS (1953). Jean Martin Charcot. In: Haymaker W, ed. *Founders of neurology*. Springfield, Charles C. Thomas:266–269.

Weinshenker BG (1995). Epidemiologic strategies to detect an exogenous cause of MS. *Acta Neurologica Scandinavica Supplementum*, 161:93–99.

Weinshenker BG et al. (1989). The natural history of multiple sclerosis: a geographically based study. I: Clinical course and disability. *Brain*, 112:133–146.

Weinshenker BG et al. (1990). A comparison of sporadic and familial multiple sclerosis. *Neurology*, 40:1354–1358.

Weitkamp LR (1983). Multiple sclerosis susceptibility. Interaction between sex and HLA. *Archives of Neurology*, 40:399–401.

Wender M, Kazmierski R (1994). The descriptive and analytical epidemiology of multiple sclerosis in western Poland. In: Firnhaber W, Lauer K, eds. *Multiple sclerosis in Europe: an epidemiological update*. Darmstadt, LTV Press:241–248.

Wender M et al. (1985). Epidemiology of multiple sclerosis in western Poland—a comparison between 1965 and 1981. *Acta Neurologica Scandinavica*, 72:210–217.

Wertman E, Zilber N, Abramsky O (1992). An association between multiple sclerosis and type I diabetes mellitus. *Journal of Neurology*, 239:43–45.

Westlund KB, Kurland LT (1953a). Studies on multiple sclerosis in Winnipeg, Manitoba, and New Orleans, Louisiana. I: Prevalence comparison between patient groups in Winnipeg and New Orleans. *American Journal of Hygiene*, 57:380–396.

Westlund KB, Kurland LT (1953b). Studies on multiple sclerosis in Winnipeg, Manitoba, and New Orleans, Louisiana. II: A controlled investigation of factors in the life history of the Winnipeg patients. *American Journal of Hygiene*, 57:397–407.

White D, Wheelan L (1959). Disseminated sclerosis: a survey of patients in Kingston, Ontario area. *Neurology*, 9:256–272.

Williams A et al. (1980). Multiple sclerosis in twins. *Neurology*, 30:1139–1147.

Williams ES, McKeran RO (1986). Prevalence of multiple sclerosis in a south London borough. *British Medical Journal (Clinical Research Edition)*, 293:237–239.

Williams ES, Jones DR, McKeran RO (1991). Mortality rates from multiple sclerosis: geographical and temporal variations revisited. *Journal of Neurology, Neurosurgery and Psychiatry*, 54:104–109.

Wolfson C, Wolfson DB, Zielinski JM (1989). On the estimation of the distribution of the latent period of multiple sclerosis. *Neuroepidemiology*, 8:239–248.

Wucherpfenning KW, Strominger JL (1995). Molecular mimicry in T cell-mediated auto-immunity: viral peptides activate human T cell clones specific for myelin basic protein. *Cell*, 80:695–705.

Wynn DR et al. (1990). A reappraisal of the epidemiology of multiple sclerosis in Olmsted County, Minnesota. *Neurology*, 40:780–786.

Yaqub BA, Daif AK (1988). Multiple sclerosis in Saudi Arabia. *Neurology*, 38:621–623.

Yu Y et al. (1989). Multiple sclerosis amongst Chinese in Hong Kong. *Brain*, 112:1445–1467.